AMBEERI SHIVAKUMAR
S.KARNAKAR REDDY

PHYTOCHEMICAL ANALYSIS OF ZINGIBER ZERUMBET (L) Roscoe ex Smith

AMBEERI SHIVAKUMAR
S.KARNAKAR REDDY

PHYTOCHEMICAL ANALYSIS OF ZINGIBER ZERUMBET (L) Roscoe ex Smith

In Vitro Propagation of Zingiber zerumbet

LAP LAMBERT Academic Publishing

Imprint
Any brand names and product names mentioned in this book are subject to trademark, brand or patent protection and are trademarks or registered trademarks of their respective holders. The use of brand names, product names, common names, trade names, product descriptions etc. even without a particular marking in this work is in no way to be construed to mean that such names may be regarded as unrestricted in respect of trademark and brand protection legislation and could thus be used by anyone.

Cover image: www.ingimage.com

Publisher:
LAP LAMBERT Academic Publishing
is a trademark of
Dodo Books Indian Ocean Ltd. and OmniScriptum S.R.L publishing group

120 High Road, East Finchley, London, N2 9ED, United Kingdom
Str. Armeneasca 28/1, office 1, Chisinau MD-2012, Republic of Moldova, Europe
Managing Directors: Ieva Konstantinova, Victoria Ursu
info@omniscriptum.com

Printed at: see last page
ISBN: 978-620-8-41683-6

CONTENT

1. INTRODUCTION

Both ancient and modern cultures have long recognized the therapeutic benefits of the compounds found in medicinal herbs. The only sources of active principles that could treat human ailments were medicinal plants and herbs until the 19th century, when chemistry and, in particular, the synthesis of organic molecules, were established. They still hold significance for those without access to contemporary medications, and both synthetic and natural pharmaceuticals today mostly depend on the same active ingredients. Because of their biodiversity, or the capacity of the plant's genetic code to create them, the active ingredients vary amongst species. There are thousands of active principles that have not yet been identified or thoroughly examined.

Medicinal plants are a worldwide legacy that originated in local custom; the world is rich in medicinal plant diversity. Because medicinal plants have been essential to maintaining human health and well-being, a comprehensive understanding of these plants for human use requires a proper scientific explanation. With nearly its entire species being edible and medicinal plants, *Zingiber* is the third biggest genus belonging to the *Zingiberaceae* family. Approx. 1200 species and 53 genera spread across South and Southeast Asia, the *Zingiberaceae* family is widely distributed (Kress et al. 2002; Khatun et al. 2003). Perennial herbs with an upright stem, aromatic odor, and fibrous rhizome characterize the plants of this genus. *Curcuma longa*, *Zingiber zerumbet*, *Zingiber officinale* and *Elettaria cardamomum* are members of this family (Andreo and Jorge, 2011).

Zingiber zerumbet (L.) Roscoe ex Smith is extensively grown throughout the world in tropical and subtropical areas (Baby et al. 2009; Madegowda et al. 2016). Bitter ginger is the common name for this species. *Z. zerumbet*, one of the major medicinal plants, is also highly significant to human medicine due to its numerous pharmacological and therapeutically useful qualities (Sahu et al. 2018).The term "Lempoyang" is exploited in Malaysia and Indonesia, "Ghatian" and "Yaiimu" in India, "Jangli adha" in Bangladesh, "Awapuhi" in Hawaii, "Zurunbah" in Arabic, "Hong qiu jiang" in China, and "Haeo dam" or "Hiao dam" in Northern Thailand, among other names. Meanwwhile, it has been grown extensively across Southeast Asia, Oceania and the Pacific, it is thought that this plant is native of India and Malaysian Peninsula.

Zingiber plants' roots are primarily utilized as culinary and medicine purpose, while the plant parts like stems, leaves, and roots are useful to extract aromatic oils. Different varieties of *Zingiber* chemical compounds were explored in recent investigations, including organic acids, volatile oils, steroids, flavonoids, terpenoids, gingerols and diarylheptanoids. A systematic evaluation of the chemical contents of the genus *Zingiber* has not been documented very often, despite the fact that many of its constituents—including some well- known ones like zerumbone, curcumin and 6-gingerol have been described (Jang et al. 2004).

1.1. Plant Profile:

Z. zerumbet is extensively grown globally, mostly in tropical and subtropical areas. *Z. zerumbet* is a smooth, upright herbaceous plant. Children with worm infections can also benefit from the usage of the boiling rhizome juice of this plant. Additionally, this can be used to treat appetite loss, sores, and edema. Because of its tendency to grow best near the base of the moist forest flora, wild ginger can form an everlasting ground cover. It needs a worm or moist, shady, rather gloomy area on the windward margins of islands where there is a lot of rainfall. It is a smooth, erect herbaceous plant with pale yellow tuberous root stocks (Prakash et al. 2011).

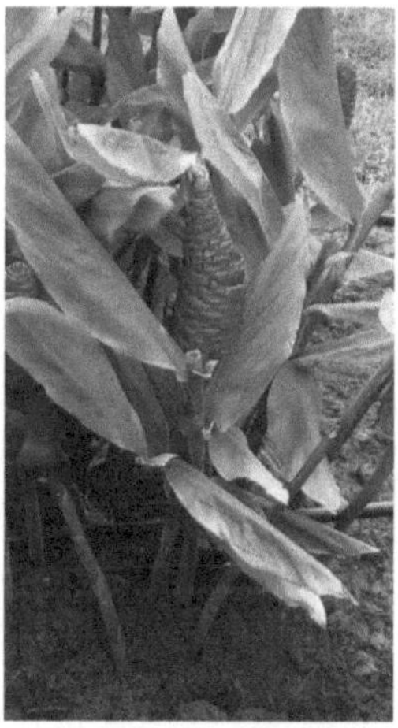

Fig. 1: The morphological appearance of *Zingiber zerumbet*

The leaf stem grows from 0.6 and 2.0 meters tall, and the leaves are arranged in the opposite way. Leaves are slender, distichous, lanceolated measuring 15 cm of length and 8 cm of width. The flowering stem that emerges straight from the root stock has a pine cone-like appearance in the late summer. The green cone becomes crimson and develops little creamy flowers on it after a few weeks. The long, appressed, obtuse sheath covering the flower stalks has an oblong-shaped or cylindrical green or crimson spike, 5 to 20 cm long, at its apex. The bracts are many, water-holding, imbricate or bicular, 2 to 3 cm long, and greenish-red in color. The fruit appears to be red oblong with 2.5 cm long; the seeds are also oblong shaped with a diameter of 4 mm. Typically, this plant has many trunks or clusters of stems (Uma and Muthukumar, 2014).

1.2. Cultivation:

Z. zerumbet is currently grown as a single rhizome or in large clusters, if provided adequate rainfall and rich organic soil, it grows swiftly. This will require regular hydration to keep the soil fairly wet, as well as full sun to light shade. The soil should have a pH of 6.1 to 6.5, which is considered somewhat acidic. Typically, clumps or portions of rhizome are divided to propagate (Stanly and Keng, 2007). This species multiplies rhizome fragments through asexual reproduction (Kavitha and Thomas, 2008).The stems of this plant are spherical, erect, oblique, and wrapped in sheaths of flat leaves. They are around 1-2 meters in height. A dense rhizome, or subterranean stem, gives rise to the leaves and inflorescences. The sheets have a pronounced raised central midrib on the lower surface, and they are thin, with a length of around 25 to 35 cm. According to Yob et al. (2011), the sheets are positioned alternating along the stem.

1.3. Taxonomical classification

Kingdom:	Plantae	Plants
Subkingdom:	Tracheobionta	Vascular plants
Superdivision:	Spermatophyta	Seed plants
Division:	Magnoliophyta	Flowering plants
Class:	Liliopsida	Monocotyledons
Subclass:	Zingiberidae	
Order:	Zingiberales	
Family:	Zingiberaceae	Ginger family
Genus:	*Zingiber* Mill.	Ginger
Species:	*Z. zerumbet* (L.) Sm.	Bitter ginger

1.4. Chemical Constituents:

Many *Zingiber* species, have rhizomes that are rich in volatile chemicals such shogaols and gingerols (Pawar et al. 2011), which are not found in *Z. zerumbet*. But *Z. zerumbet*'s unique flavor, scent, and therapeutic ability are due to possesion of its crucial bioactive ingredients, including zerumbone, curcuminoids, and other oleoresins (Koga et al. 2016). Zerumbone, a primary constituent of *Z. zerumbet* is a monocyclic sesquiterpene with a significant antitumoral molecule (Kitayama, 2011; Padalia et al. 2018). The pharmaceutical and cosmeceutical sectors have high demand for it (Murakami et al. 2002). Furthermore, zerumbone was discovered to have chemopreventive properties against hepato-carcinogenesis (Taha et al. 2010).

A class of biologically active polyphenolic substances called curcuminoids is frequently utilized as food additives and coloring agents. They include curcumin, demethoxycurcumin, and bisdemethoxycurcumin (Sathishkumar et al. 2015). These substances, which are mostly found in *Z. zerumbet*, have demonstrated a variety of biological and pharmacological activities (Chan et al. 2023). *Z. zerumbet* is abundant source of various chemicals, including alkaloids, polyphenols and terpenes that correspond to a broad range of chemical metabolites (Murthy et al. 2022). According to Yob et al. (2011), phytochemical analyses of the plant demonstrated that the rhizomes are rich source of flavonoids, phenolics, and numerous sesquiterpenoids. High levels of phenolic chemicals are thought to give the plant several biological benefits, including strong antioxidant activity (Ghasemzadeh et al. 2016). Ramaswami and Bhattacharyya (1962) identified humulene dioxide and monoxide, whereas Dev (1960) extracted zerumbone from *Z. zerumbet* essential oil and found its structure. Following a study by Nigam and Levi (1963), the following chemicals were identified: borneol, camphor, α-caryophyllene, α-humulene, linalool, limonene, α-pinene, and zerumbone. The following sesquiterpenes were described by Damodaran and Dev (1968): caryophyllene oxide, humulene epoxide (I, II, III) and humulenol (I, II).

Dai et al. (2013) report that suggested that the essential oils isolated from *Z. zerumbet*'s rhizome included 46 different components. Monoterpenes, including citral, *Zingiber*ene, camphene, sabinene, and lavandulyl acetate, were the most prevalent constituents. The essential oil in the aforementioned investigation has a low level of zerumbone. Zerumbone is monocyclic sesquiterpene that has 3 double bonds: one is isolated, while the other two are connected with carbonyl groups (Kitayama, 2011; Padalia et al.

2018). Zerumbone was quantitatively analyzed by Rout et al. (2009) in several *Z. zerumbet* locations. The roots had the lowest values, and the rhizome had the highest.

1.5. Traditional uses

It is commonly acknowledged that there is a need for confirmation on the widely held notion that medicinal plants can be deployed for treating various illnesses. The customary application of therapeutic plants aids in the dissemination of this understanding and provides a foundation for investigations by scientists looking for proof of these pharmacological actions. The portion of *Z. zerumbet* most frequently utilized for medicinal reasons is the rhizome (Norulaini et al. 2009). Generally, fresh rhizome is macerated and infusion-prepared to create these traditional remedies, but alternative medicinal applications include tinctures, poultices, and even the plant itself (Tushar et al. 2010).

Furthermore to its numerous traditional applications, *Z. zerumbet* possesses pharmacological and biological qualities. The long-lasting cone-shaped flowers are used as ornaments in craft arrangements (Devi et al. 2014).The rhizome has stimulating and tonic properties (Sakinah et al. 2007). Whereas the flower buds were used as vegetables, the rhizome as flavoring in food (Sirirugsa, 1999).With remarkable therapeutic results, ginger rhizome has been widely used to treat bacterial infections, inflammation, diarrhea, cramps in the stomach, fever, flatulence, allergies, and poisoning (Sidahmed et al. 2015; Chan et al. 2023).

The rhizome powder is used to relieve toothaches, ear infections, and stomach illnesses when brewed as tea (Ghosh et al. 2011). Additionally, the leaves were used to treat joint pains. Children's worm infestations have reportedly been successfully treated with the juice of boiled rhizome (Somchit and Shukriyah, 2003; Tandon et al. 2011). Rich in surfactants, the creamy material found in mature inflorescences functions as natural shampoo (Nalawade et al. 2003).

1.6. Pharmacological Properties

Z. zerumbet rhizomes essential oil has been extensively researched due to its great medicinal potential and application in perfumes. It is enriched with different active aromatic metabolites (Chavan and Dey, 2023). Rhizome oil contains large amounts of zerumbone, a monocyclic sesquiterpenoid ($C_{15}H_{22}O$) with pharmacological and biological properties like anti-inflammatory, anti-proliferative and antioxidant effects (Singh et al. 2019). Zerumbone's anticancer effect, which it provides by inhibiting the stimulation of gene expression produced by carcinogens and preventing cancer cells from undergoing apoptosis, has made it extremely important (Girisa et al. 2019). According to bioassay research, zerumbone largely inhibits the growth of many cancer types while having little impact on healthy cells (Abdelwahab et al. 2012; Rahman et al. 2014).

1.7. Insecticidal properties

Essential oils extracted from the plants belonging to the Zingiberaceae family are toxic to insects (Suthisut et al. 2011; Madreseh-Ghahfarokhi et al. 2018; Keosaeng et al. 2023). Fresh rhizomes from *Z. zerumbet* and *Curcuma zedoaria,* native to southern Thailand, are used in Thai cuisine. Moreover, *Zingiber* genus essential oils have exhibited properties like anticancer (Soumya et al. 2023), antibacterial (Sharifi-Rad et al. 2017), antifungal (ALFahdawi and Joudah, 2020), and anti-inflammatory (Paramita et al. 2021).

1.8. Tissue culture studies in medicinal plants

Scientific cultivation and conservation efforts are necessary due to overexploitation, which goes well beyond the natural potential for regeneration caused by declining populations. Specifically, rapid multiplication strategy needs to be established for sustainable farming and conservation (Sharmin et al. 2014). Tissue culture, or *in vitro* propagation, can quickly multiply the rate to solve the problems and aid in conservation, cultivation, and propagation that is sustainable (Anis and Ahmad, 2016). Micropropagation provides true-to- type, uniform offsprings with respect to its end products, such as the bioactive chemicals. Additionally, it is desirable to preserve germplasm (from healthy meristems) *in vitro* since it requires less space and labor and prevents the accumulation of infections and mutations (Alam et al. 2013).

1.8.1. In vitro propagation of Z. zerumbet

Owing to its many health advantages, this herb merits particular consideration and a wider cultural dissemination. According to this view, biotechnological applications particularly in plant tissue culture play an important role for regeneration of true to type, prolific, disease free, *Z. zerumbet* clones in large scale. While, genetic influence over morphological and biochemical properties is a major problem with the production of aromatic and medicinal plants using tissue culture for producing quality and stable crude medicines (Pant, 2014). To overcome this complexity, it is critical to evaluate the drug-producing potential of the clones that were developed *in vitro* as well as in field conditions to determine the efficacy of the drug-producing characteristics.

Rhizomes are the conventional method of propagating *Z. zerumbet.* Since fungi can cause diseases that impair the quality of the tubers, the rhizome should not be kept in storage for extended periods of time (Nalawade et al. 2003). As a result, micropropagation presents itself as a viable substitute technique for growing vast quantities of homogeneous, pathogen-free plants with high-quality rhizomes (Poonsapaya and Krasintu, 1993). Nalawade et al. (2003) report demonstrated that the deployment of plant tissue culture technique for safe exchange of germplasm across international borders with the aim to produce numerous free of pathogens, identical and elite clones, uncommon, and essential native medicinal plants for restoration in their natural habitats.

By mimicking the *in vivo* ambient environment through aseptic tissue culture, the approach promotes growth and development while maintaining the integrity of plant both structurally and functionally. The utilization of tissue culture approach for plant regeneration is urgently needed in horticulture and agriculture, given the economic value of the target plant variety (Gulzar et al. 2020). Potential methods for generating quality plants by tissue culture-based genetic improvement initiatives of progenies that are clonaly selected, mutation bred, and polyploidy induced (Debnath et al. 2020). Because of its great commercial importance, a variety of *in vitro* regeneration techniques have been improved using nutritional supplementation, plant growth regulators and various environmental parameters that govern cellular growth and development (Bidabadi and Jain, 2020).

The development and optimization of *in vitro* regeneration protocol for specific plant types has led to rapid establishment of tissue culture facilities. This has produced high-value metabolites, disease-free plant varieties, successful plant multiplication, and *ex vitro* germplasm conservation, demonstrating its role in lessening the encumbrance on farmers (Debnath et al. 2020). Overall crop improvement also benefited from large-scale propagation techniques and *in vitro* regeneration under *Zingiber*-optimized environments. Consequently, all of these initiatives have improved the synthesis of secondary metabolites and medicinal molecules.

1.8.2. Studies on genetic variations

Z. zerumbet's phytochemicals have been thoroughly investigated. Several investigations have reported on *Z. zerumbet* rhizome-based *in vitro* plant regeneration. Although, this method is not appropriate to true to type plantlets, rhizome bud culture for induction of *in vitro* shoots still needs to be improved for rapid multiplication, and most importantly, genetic homogeneity testing among the plantlets (Rakkimuthu et al. 2011; Victório et al. 2011). Furthermore, as genotype influences *in vitro* culture responses, evaluations of transplants from various geographic locations are required in order to propose a broadly applicable procedure. There are no reports on DNA-based identification or testing homogeneity among plants grown in tissue cultures. In particular, the genus gingiber needs to establish DNA markers in order to more clearly define its genertc boundary (Kress et al. 2002). The current work aims to determine molecular identity of the species and create a successful micropropagation strategy backed by genetic fidelity based on DNA markers. These would be helpful in cultivation and conservation methods as well as in precisely identifying the therapeutic plant for the phytomedicine sector.

Medicinal plants often exhibit significant intraspecific variation with respect to a range of phytochemical profile (Azizi, 2010). True-to-type plantlets and genetic stability are key components of micropropagation commercially, which led to physiological as well as soma clonal heterogeneity, since *in vitro* produced plant cell, tissue, organ and undifferentiated calli are often associated with genetic modifications during the process (Bidabadi and Jain, 2020). Variation in *in vitro* propagated plants is governed by the source of the explant or plant regeneration procedure. Both genetic and epigenetic factors can cause somaclonal variations; these include genotype, the chimeras, the kind and provenance of explants, the media type, plant growth regulators range, culture duration and culture environment (temperature and light) (Kaçar, 2024).

The wide range of applications for micropropagation systems may be restricted by these factors. While soma clonal diversity helps in the selection of novel genotypes, it is harmful to the preservation of germplasm, so in order to maintain different genotypes, these elite genotypes must be multiplied. When creating conservation programs, evaluating genetic diversity and purity is essential. Genetic, morphological, physiological, and biochemical analyses could all be deployed to verify the homogeneity of *in vitro* grown plants (Bidabadi and Jain, 2020). As DNA-based markers were not impacted by environmental factors, they offer a promising means of verifying the clonal fidelity of tissue culture plants.

Genetic fidelity studies employ PCR-based DNA markers, including sequence-based (Simple Sequence Repeat, SSR) and semi-arbitrary (Inter-Simple Sequence Repeat, ISSR; Amplified Fragment Length Polymorphism, and AFLP) approaches (Singh et al. 2012). RAPD markers are prominently utilized for genetic affinity analysis due to their capacity to amplify a wide range of genomic regions. RAPD and ISSR analysis revealed that no genetic variation was observed in plants derived from callus compared to the donar plant. This suggests that these protocols can be used for large scale and true-to-type propagation of identical plantlets in *C. caesia* (Jose and Thomas, 2015). Several regenerated plantlets from the *Zingiber*aceae family, including *Alpinia calcarata*, are being cultivated *in vitro*, and ISSR technology is being utilized to assess their genetic integrity (Das et al. 2016).

1.8.3. Advantages of Micropropagation:

Compared to conventional propagation method, micropropagation offers a number of benefits, such as rapid multiplication and disease-free plants (Gupta et al. 2020). Thus, elite genotypes of *Zingiber* species that are extremely vulnerable to different illnesses can be generated via *in vitro* micropropagation methods (Chakraborty et al., 2023). The two main methods for achieving plant micropropagation *in vitro* are callus formation and direct organogenesis. Calli cultures generated from *in vitro* explants can be useful for production organs like shoots, roots, storage organs *via* the de-differentiation process. Using auxiliary buds as explants to cultivate apical meristematic tissue is another approach to generate *in vitro* plants.

It is likely that *in vitro* plants are disease free and the meristematic cells also facilitate growth of the plant and develop the different plant parts. This method also has the benefit of avoiding callus development and adventitious organogenesis, as organs produced directly from meristematic cells, safeguarding the genetic stability and reducing somaclonal variation (Haque et al. 2022). Somatic embryogenesis, which creates embryo from a single cell and results in full plant growth, is another technique utilized in micropropagation. This technique could be rapid and effective strategy to propagate on wide scale with reduced multiplication period since it exploits the embryogenic route *in vitro* (Kumar and Reddy, 2011).

The primary goal of this study was to comprehensively examine *Z. zerumbet* and develop an efficient *in vitro* propagation technique for it. Through molecular characterisation, critical phytochemical identification, and validation of these phytochemicals against a variety of plant pathogenic bacteria, fungus, and insect pests, our work maintains genetic integrity. These findings foster environmentally friendly and sustainable farming methods by opening the door to *Z. zerumbet's* commercial cultivation and utilization in an array of industries.

1.9. Objectives

- To establish *in vitro* regeneration method from rhizome explants of *Zingiber zerumbet.*
- To evaluate the genetic fidelity of *in vitro* regenerated plantlets of *Z. zerumbet* using RAPD molecular markers.
- To investigate the phytochemical analysis of *Z. zerumbet* rhizome extracts quantitatively and qualitatively by GC-MS.
- To evaluate the antagonistic effect of *Z. zerumbet* rhizome extracts on plant pathogenic bacteria, fungi and insect pest.

2. MATERIALS AND METHOD

2.1.1. Plant material and chemicals:

Plant seed of *Zingiber* zerumbet was obtained from Telangana State Agricultural University, Rajendranagar, Hyderabad, thanks to Prof. Jayashanker. Unless indicated differently, all compounds were analytical grade and were procured from Sisco Research Laboratories or HiMedia in Mumbai, India. Sigma-Aldrich supplied the agar, and plant growth regulators.

2.1.2. Collection and surface sterilization of explant:

Rhizomes of *Zingiber zerumbet* were collected and maintained in a plot. The sprouting rhizomes were collected (Fig. 2a) and washed under continuous running water and then washed with detergent to remove any residues of soil. The bud parts of rhizomes were excised, trimmed and performed sterilization using bavistin (5 g/L), tween 20 (few drops) subsequently, sterile distilled water was used to rinse the explants. Additional surface sterilization was performed using laminar air flow, the rhizome bud explants were disinfected at varied time periods (5, 10, and 15 minutes) using varying concentrations of NaOCl (5% and 10% v/v) and C_2H_5OH (50 and 70% v/v). The rhizome bud explants were then washed 3 times with SDW. Followed by treatment with 0.1% (w/v) $HgCl_2$ for 5, 10, and 15 minutes, the transplants were rinsed five times with SDW to remove any remaining harmful effects from the sterilants.

2.1.3. Pre-culture of rhizome explants:

The 200 ml screw-capped culture bottles were inoculated with one sterile rhizome explant that contained 30 ml of Basal MS (Murashige and Skoog, 1962) media that contained 0.8% (w/v) agar and 3% sucrose (Fig. 2b). Before adding agar, the medium's pH was adjusted to 5.8 with 1 N NaOH or HCl. It was then autoclaved for 15 minutes at 121 °C. After repeatedly washing the explants in sterile distilled water, they were kept for air drying on sterile tissue paper under a flow and inoculated on medium.

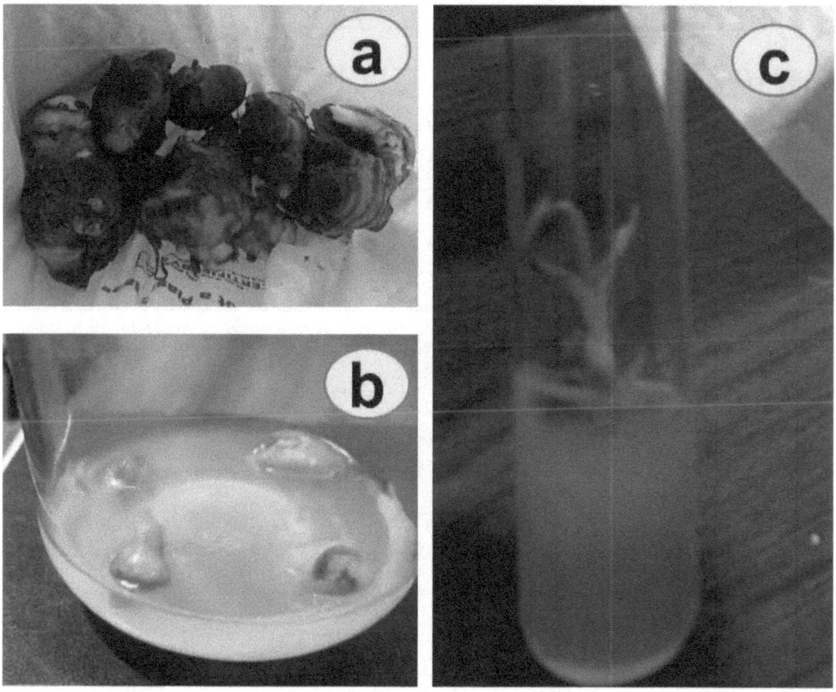

Fig. 2. Detailed picture of *Z. zerumbet* sample collected **(a),** surface sterilized explant incoculated **(b),** and healthy sprouted rhizome bud **(c).**

Table. 1. Tabular form of Morishige and Skoog Media composition

Components Name	Concentration (mg/L)	Weight (mg)
Macronutrients	**1x**	**10x**
KNO_3	1900	19000
NH_4NO_3	1650	16500
$MgSO_4.\ 7H_2O$	370	3700
$CaCl_2.\ 2H_2O$	440	4400
KH_2PO_4	170	1700
Micronutrients		
Minor B	**1x**	**500x (100 ml)**
H_3BO_3	6.2	310
$NaMoO_4.\ 2H_2O$	0.25	12.5
$CoCl_2.\ 6H_2O$	0.025	1.25
KI	0.83	41.5
Minor C	**1x**	**500x (100 ml)**
$MnSO_4.\ 4H_2O$	22.3	1115
$ZnSO_4.\ 7H_2O$	8.6	430
$CuSO_4.\ 5H_2O$	0.025	1.25
Minor D	**1x**	**500x (100 ml)**
$FeSO_4.\ 7H_2O$	27.8	1390
Na_2EDTA	37.3	1865
Minor E	**1x**	**500x (100 ml)**
Thiamine hydrochloride	0.1	5
Pyridoxine hydrochloride	0.5	25
Nicotinic acid	0.5	25
Glycine	2	100
Minor F		
Myo inositol	100	1000

2.1.4. Shoot bud multiplication medium:

Using KN (0.2, 0.4, 0.6, 0.8, and 1.0 mg/L) and NAA (0.4 mg/L), the sprouted rhizome bud explants (Fig. 2d) were inoculated on the medium and allowed to incubate for a whole week. Following the addition of KN (0.4 mg/L) and NAA (0.4 mg/L) to the MS medium, on which the explants were subcultured, BAP was added at varying concentrations (1, 2, 3, 4, and 5 mg/l). To enhance the quantity of shoots, TDZ was supplemented to the medium above at varied concentrations (1, 2, 3, 4, and 5 mg/L). The MS basal medium as described by Murashige and Skoog (1962) (Table 1), 30 g/L sucrose supplement was added to the medium. Subsequently, the medium was then autoclaved at 121 °C, 15 lbs pressure for 20 minutes, and its pH was corrected to 5.8 after being solidified with 8 g/L agar. A cool fluorescent light with a photosynthetic flux of 150 µmol m^{-2} s^{-1} and a 16-hour photoperiod were used to maintain all cultures at 25 ± 2 °C.

2.1.5. *In vitro* rooting and elongation:

Individual shoots of ~3.20 cm length were separated from the shoot clusters after the multiplication stage and placed onto MS medium fortified with different concentrations of indole-3-butyric acid (IBA, 0.5, 1.0, 1.5, and 2.0 mg/l), either by themselves or in conjunction with BA (2 mg/l) or KN (2 mg/l). The cultures were maintained for three weeks in standard culture conditions, which included a 16-hour photoperiod and 64 µE/m^2/s of white fluorescent light emission.

2.1.6. Acclimatization:

Once the plantlets developed roots, they were removed carefully from the medium and washed thoroughly under running water to get rid of the clinging solid MS medium. They were then moved into plastic pots filled with sterile peat moss soil and transferred into the net house that offered 50% shade. Transparent perforated polyethylene bags were used to cover the plants in order to keep the humidity high and avoid plant dryness from water loss. To keep the humidity high, the plants were regularly watered. The plastic bags were removed after 15 days, and the plantlets were given a further two weeks to acclimate.

2.1.7. Collection of data:

After completion of 8 weeks of culture, the following metrics were assessed: the quantity of roots and branches as well as their length.

2.1.8. Genomic DNA isolation:

The whole genomic DNA of the donar plant and the *in vitro* reproduced plants was extracted independently from the fresh leaves using a Cetyl trimethyl ammonium bromide (CTAB) method. Doyle & Doyle provided a description of this process (1987). DNA was quantified at 260 nm and the 260/280 nm ratio was used to assess the purity. The PCR reactions were performed in a total volume of 25 µl including template DNA (25 ng), primer (5 pM), 10X reaction buffer containing 15 mM $MgCl_2$, 200 M of each dNTP, and 3U/µl of Taq polymerase.

For the purpose of amplifying genomic DNA, a thermal cycler with the following programming was utilized: After 5 minutes of initial heating at 94 °C, there are 40 cycles of 1 min of denaturation at 94 °C, 1 minute of annealing at 35 °C, 2 minutes of extension at 72 °C, and 7 min of final extension at 72 °C. Gel documentation system (BioRad, CA, USA) was used to capture the image of the amplified reaction products were separated electrophoretically on a 1.5% agarose gel stained with 0.5 g/ml ethidium bromide and seen under ultraviolet light.

2.1.9. RAPD analysis:

Different random primers were used to assess Z. *Zingiber*'s genetic variation each variety's PCR was conducted using the same concentration of DNA. An Eppendorf Master Cycler PCR Machine (Hamburg, Germany) was used to conduct RAPD reactions. 2 µl of 10X PCR buffer (MBI Fermentas, Vilnius, Lithuania), 0.5 µl of 10 mM dNTP (deoxyribonucleotide triphosphate, MBI Fermentas), 2 µl of 10 picomoles/µl primer (Bioserve, Hyderabad, India), 15 ng of template DNA, 0.2 µl of Taq polymerase (5U/µl, MBI Fermentas), and sterile milli-Q water were included in the 20 µl reaction mixture. 42 cycles of amplification and final extension at 72 °C for 5 min were followed by holding the amplified products at 4 °C. The PCR amplification process involved pre-denaturation at 94 °C for 3 min, denaturation at 94 °C for 30 sec, primer annealing at 40 °C for 1 min and primer extension at 72 °C for 2 min. Following PCR completion, the amplified products were separated on 1.2% agarose gel in 1X Tris-acetate solution at 100V for two hours. 6X loading dye was then added to the PCR product. DNA was seen using a UV transilluminator (UVitec, Cambridge, U.K.) after being stained with ethidium bromide (0.5 mg/l, Sigma, St. Louis, U.S.A.). The Gel Documentation System (Syngene, Frederick, U.S.A.) was used to scan the gel pictures. The DNA ladder, which ranges from 100 to 3000 bp (MBI Fermentas, Vilnius, Lithuania), was used to estimate the band sizes.

2.1.10. Statistical analysis:

The Sigma Plot software, version 12, was used to analyse the collected data. To compare the means of various treatments, analysis of variance (ANOVA) with mean deviation by Holms-Sidak ($P<0.05$) was utilized. Triplicates of each experiment was conducted.

2.2.1. Preparation of plant extracts:

After *Z. zerumbet* was collected, the rhizomes of the harvested plants were separated and identified. After mature rhizomes were allowed to air dry for 72 hours, 2.5 g of powdered dry matter and 25 mL of solvent were magnetically stirred for 30 minutes at room temperature (25°C) to extract plant extracts. Acetone/water (8:2, v/v), ethanol/water (8:2, v/v), hexane (8:2, v/v), methanol/water (8:2, v/v) and water were the solvents used to create the extracts, which had varying degrees of polarity. After being held at 4°C for a full day, the extract was filtered using Whatman No. 4 filter paper, vacuum-dried to a dry state, and then kept at 4°C until analysis.

2.2.2. Determination of total soluble protein:

Total soluble protein was measured using bovine serum albumin (BSA) at 640 nm as a standard, following Lowry's 1951 method. The 100 mg of dry rhizome powder samples was ground finely in 10 mM ice cold potassium phosphate buffer (pH 6.8) and centrifuged for 20 minutes at 15,000 g. The amount of soluble protein was ascertained using the resulting supernatant. The units of measurement were mg per g of fresh weight (FW).

2.2.3. Total flavonoids estimation:

The aluminum chloride method for estimation of the total flavonoid content was followed as described by Dewanto et al. (2002). After being suspended in 10 milliliters of 80% methanol for 24 h at room temperature, a total of 250 mg of the powdered sample was centrifuged for 20 minutes at 3000 rpm. The supernatant extract was removed from the test tubes, containing 1.0 ml. After adding 0.3 ml of a 5% $NaNO_2$ solution, this was left for three minutes. 0.3 ml of 10% $AlCl_3$ was added after three minutes, and the mixture was left for two minutes. After adding 2 ml of 1.0 M NaOH, thoroughly mix, 2.4 ml of distilled water was then added, and everything was thoroughly mixed. The golden brown color's optical density was measured at 510 nm. Using the quercitine standard curve as a guide, the total flavonoid content was computed and reported as mg/g dry weight.

2.2.4. Total phenolic content estimation:

In accordance with Dewanto et al. (2002), total phenols were tested. A portion of the diluted extract was added to 0.125 mL of Folin-Ciocalteu reagent and 0.5 mL of distilled water in an aliquot. 1.25 mL of 7% Na_2CO_3 was added after the mixture was agitated and left for 6 min. Following a thorough mixing, the solution's ultimate volume of 3 mL was adjusted with distilled water. Upon dark incubation, absorbance at 760 nm was measured in comparison with blank. The total phenol content of plant parts was measured using a calibration curve with gallic acid and represented as milligrams of gallic acid equivalents per gram of dry weight (mg GAE/g DW). Three duplicates of each sample were examined.

2.2.5. Estimation of total condensed tannins:

The Sun et al. (1998) method was used to quantify the amount of condensed tannins, also known as proanthocyanidins. 1.5 mL of concentrated HCl and 3 mL of 4% vanillin solution in methanol was added to 50 μL of diluted sample. After 15 min of incubation, the reaction mixture's absorbance was read at 500 nm using methanol as a blank. The unit of measurement for total condensed tannin content is mg (+)-catechin/g DW. Every sample was examined three times.

2.2.6. DPPH assay:

Using the Hanato et al. (1988) method, the extracted materials' capacity to donate electrons was assessed by bleaching a purple solution containing 1,1-diphenyl-2-picrylhydrazyl (DPPH) radical. 0.5 mL of a 0.2 μmol/L DPPH methanol solution was mixed with extracts (1, 5, 10, 50, and 100μg/mL). Following a 30 min incubation period at room temperature, the absorbance at 517 nm was recorded in comparison to a blank. The formula for calculating the percentage of inhibition of free radical DPPH was (A blank−A sample/A blank) × 100, where A blank represents the absorbance of the control reaction and A sample represents the absorbance of plant extract. The regression equation for the concentration of extract and percentage of inhibition was used to ascertain the concentration of extract that induced 50% inhibition (IC50). The samples underwent triplicate analysis.

2.2.7. Total antioxidant capacity:

The assay is based on the extract's reduction of Mo(VI) to Mo(V) and the consequent formation of a green phosphate–Mo(V) complex at an acid pH (Prieto (1999). An aliquot (0.1 mL) of plant extract was mixed with 1 mL of the reagent (0.6 mol/L H_2SO_4, 28 mmol/L Na_3PO_4 and 4 mmol/L ammonium molybdate). The vials were incubated in a thermal block for 90 minutes at 95°C. The mixture was cooled to room temperature, the absorbance of each solution was recorded at 695 nm relative to a blank. Gallic acid equivalent per gram of dry weight, or milligrams (mg GAE/g DW), was used to quantify the antioxidant ability. The calibration curve's range was 0–500 ꞁg/mL. Each sample underwent three examinations.

2.2.8. Gas chromatography/mass spectrometry (GC/MS) analysis:

2.2.8.1. GC-MS analysis:

Using GC-MS SHIMADZU GCMSQP2010, the components of *Z. zerumbet* rhizome extract were identified. The employed column had an inner diameter of 30 m × 0.25 mm and 0.25 μm thickness. Helium was used as carrier gas (flow rate: 1 mL/min), at a rate of 4 ◦C per minute, the oven temperature was raised to 300 ◦C while the injector temperature was maintained at 280 ◦C. The identification was performed using the NIST library in accordance with the accepted practices outlined in Padalia et al. (2013)'s earlier papers.

2.3.1. Collection of microorganisms:

The antibacterial activity was performed against two Gram (-) ve bacteria (*Xanthomonas spp* and *Pseudomonas syringae*). The screening of antifungal activity was carried out against three fungi (*Rhizoctonia solani, Fusarium oxysporum* and *Colletotrichum capsici*). All these organisms were collected from the Crop Protection and Biological Control Laboratory, SLN Biologicals LLP, Nizamabad, Telangana, India.

2.3.2. Collection of test insect:

The experimental Aphids (*Aphis gossypii*) were obtained from stock cultures at the Crop Protection and Biological Control Laboratory, SLN Biologicals LLP, Nizamabad, Telangana, India, for the purpose of insecticidal screening.

2.3.3. Growth media and conditions:

For antibacterial and antifungal screening, HiMedia Laboratories' nutrient agar medium (pH 7.2) and potato dextrose agar medium (pH 5.6) were utilized, respectively.

2.3.4. Antibacterial screening:

The disc diffusion method was used to examine the extract's in vitro antibacterial activity (Bauer et al. 1996). Each sterile disc of 6 mm in diameter was made up of filter paper was allowed to absorb 20 µl of a sample solution in order to create sample discs. The discs were left to dry out until all of the solvent was evaporated. Filter paper discs that had been dried and sterilized, 500 µg of the test agent was placed on nutrient agar medium that had been evenl y seeded with the test microorganisms. The positive and negative controls were a blank disc and a kanamycin disc (30 µg/disc), respectively. For 24 hours, the plates were incubated at 37° C to promote the best possible growth for the organisms. The zone of inhibition diameter was expressed in millimeters and it is used to calculate the extract's antibacterial activity.

2.3.5. Antifungal screening:

The disc diffusion method was used to screen the extract for antifungal activity at a 500µg/disc concentration. Potato dextrose (20 ml) plates were prepared and aseptically incubated using the spread plate method. Using sterile forceps, the impregnated discs containing plant extract was placed on the agar and carefully pressed down to ensure full contact between the disc and the surface. Carbendezim control discs were made and put on the agar surface. Following a 72-hour incubation period at 37°C, the dimensions of the inhibitory zones were measured on each plate. The plant extract's mean zone of inhibition for the three replicated experiments (triplicate study) is given in millimeters.

2.3.6. Insecticidal screening:

Test tubes were obtained for the plant extract's surface film activity test. The 500 mg of plant extract was dissolved in 1 ml of methanol and then mixed with 10 ml of sterile water that contained 5 percent sucrose. This was added to the lower section of the petridish. At the same time, standard conditions was set at 28 °C, 70% relative humidity and a photoperiod of 12 h of light and 12 h of darkness. For control experiment, water alone was added to the test tube slants (Bousquet, 1990). Following the completion of all preparations, treated petridishes were kept at room temperature and kept safe. Periodically, the entire experiment was observed, and data was compiled on mortality after 24, 48, and 72 h of exposure. Using a basic microscope, the insects were observed by following their natural movements. To verify death, a hot needle was occasionally brought closer to their bodies without causing any movement.

2.3.7. Statistical analysis:

The one way ANOVA was deployed to statistically analyze the data, and SigmaPlot version 12.0 was used to evaluate significant difference among the treatments using Duncan's multiple range test (DMRT) at the $P = 0.05$ level. The EPA Probit analysis program (1.5) was used to perform probability analysis for the purpose of LC50 value computation. The LogProbit analysis was used to get the inhibition ratio and EC50 values.

3. RESULTS

3.1. Establishment of micropropagation method and to evaluate the genetic stability of micropropagated plantlets of *Z. zerumbet* 's using RAPD molecular markers

Plant tissue culture or *in vitro* propagation, is a method that facilitates the large scale multiplication of plants under controlled and sterile conditions. This method is particularly advantageous for species like *Zingiber zerumbet*, where traditional propagation through rhizomes can be slow and inefficient. *In vitro* propagation from rhizome explants not only accelerates the production of healthy and uniform plantlets but also facilitates the conservation of valuable genetic material and supports commercial cultivation efforts.

3.1.1. Selection of explants:

The initial step in the *in vitro* propagation of *Zingiber zerumbet* involves the selection of appropriate explants. Rhizomes are the preferred explants due to their rich source of meristematic tissues, which are capable of regenerating new shoots. Healthy, disease-free rhizomes are carefully chosen for the process (Fig. 2a). The establishment of explants *in vitro* can be attributed by several factors, one of which is surface sterilization, which can be accomplished using a variety of sterilizing chemicals to combat microbial contamination.

3.1.2. Surface sterilization:

Various sterilizing chemicals were used in our investigation to maximize surface sterilization during establishment of *in vitro* cultures using rhizome explants collected from the field (Fig. 2a). Usually, these rhizomes are surface-sterilized with a series of sterilants such ethanol, sodium hypochlorite, or mercuric chloride. To eliminate any contaminants, a thorough rinse with sterile distilled water is then performed. Among the many sterilizing agents evaluated the study's rhizome buds were sterilized using $HgCl_2$ (0.1%) for 2 min. Following 3 rounds of washing with sterile distilled water, the microorganisms with the highest *in vitro* culture establishment were eradicated (Fig. 2d).

3.1.3. Pre-culture of explants:

After sterilization, the rhizome explants are dissected into small segments, typically 1-2 cm in length, containing at least one dormant bud. Following that, these sterilized explants are cultures under aseptic conditions on an appropriate nutrient medium. Murashige and Skoog (MS) media (Table 1) is most widely used medium for *Zingiber zerumbet* propagation. It is enriched with different growth regulators, like cytokinins (e.g., BAP - 6-

benzylaminopurine) for promoting shoot regeneration. The explants are grown in a growth chamber with highly controlled temperatures (around 25–28°C), light (16-hour photoperiod), and humidity. Within a few weeks, the rhizome explants typically begin to produce multiple shoots, a process known as shoot induction.

In the given study also, after one week of pre-culturing the surface-sterilized explants on basal media, considerable changes were observed in the percentage of the explants that survived and sprouted (Fig. 2d).

3.1.4. Shoot multiplication:

Once the initial shoots emerge, they can be subcultured to fresh media to promote further multiplication. The multiplication phase involves repeated cycles of transferring the growing shoots to new culture media, enriched with appropriate concentrations of cytokinins, to stimulate the production of additional shoots. This step is crucial for generating a more number of plantlets from a single explant. During this phase, the concentration of growth regulators can be modified, and other supplements, such as auxins (e.g., NAA - naphthalene acetic acid), may be added to enhance shoot elongation and vigor. Regular subculturing every 3-4 weeks ensures continuous and exponential shoot proliferation.

In this study, the *Z. zerumbet* rhizome bud explants grown on MS media fortified with varying concentrations of KN (0.2, 0.4, 0.6, 0.8, and 1.0 mg/L) and NAA (0.4 mg/L), on which both shoots and roots concurrently generated, with shoot induction being the lowest (2.00). Explants were subcultured on MS media containing BAP (1, 2, 3, 4, and 5 mg/l) in conjunction with NAA (0.4 mg/L) and KN (0.4 mg/L), which resulted in increased shoot quantity and length (Table. 2) (Fig. 3d). In this study, the inclusion of 1 mg/L BAP, 2 mg/L TDZ and 0.4 mg/L NAA in the medium to increase the shoot multiplication (Table. 2).

The highest shoot number was noticed in MS media supplemented with 1.0 mg/L BAP, 2 mg/L TDZ and 0.4 mg/L NAA (Fig. 3f). Number of shoots and shoot length per explant augmented at all BAP concentrations. As a result, it indicates that BAP has a beneficial influence on *Z. zerumbet* shoot multiplication *in vitro*. The proliferating shoots appeared green and robust. In the given study also, the inclusion of 1 mg/L BAP, 2 mg/L TDZ and 0.4 mg/L NAA in the medium increased the number of proliferating shoots (20.00) significantly (Table. 2).

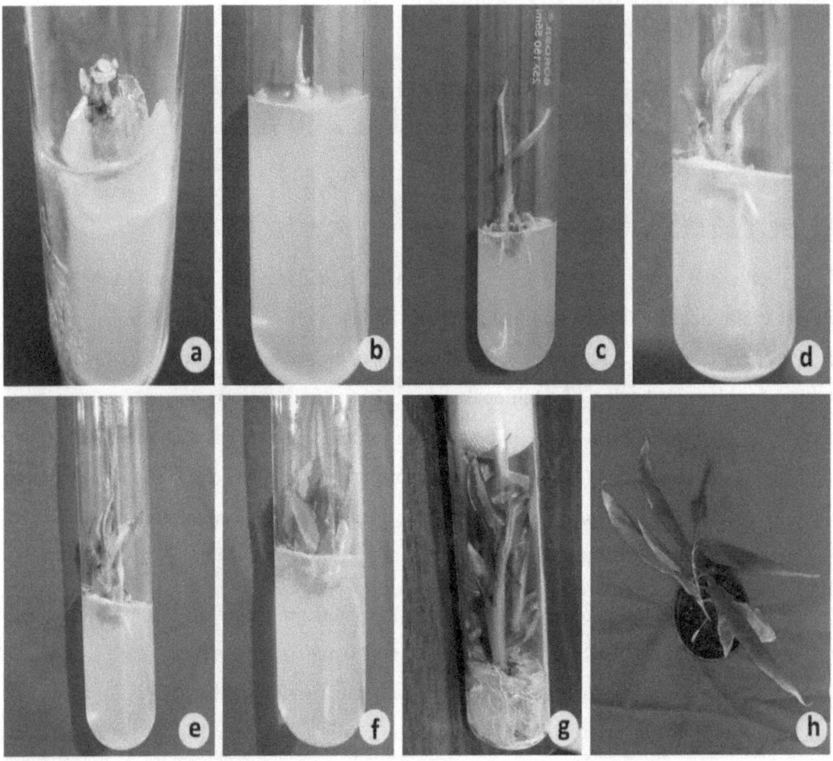

Fig. 3. Various stages of the *Z. zerumbet* rhizome explants' *in vitro* regeneration. (a) Inoculation of rhizome bud explants on MS medium containing different concentrations of KN (0.2-1.0 mg/L) + NAA (0.4 mg/L); (b) Sprouted explant; (c) Sprout elongation; (d) Subculture on to the medium containing BAP (1-5 mg/L), KN (0.4 mg/L), NAA (0.4 mg/L);
(e) Responding with 3-4 shoots per explant; (f) Sub-culture on to the medium containing TDZ (2 mg/L), BAP (1 mg/L), NAA (0.4 mg/L); (g) Rooting of multiplied explants on MS media containing NAA (1 mg/L); (h) Hardening of *in vitro* raised plantlet of *Z. zerumbet.*

3.1.5. Induction of *in vitro* roots from regenerated shoots:

In vitro rooting was induced on MS medium fortified with IBA and NAA, the number of roots was varied with varying IBA or NAA concentrations. On an average, 31 roots were induced per shoot especially with 1 mg/l NAA at an average root length of 2.73 cm, while IBA at 1 mg/l induced 11.66 roots with an mean root length of 2.96 cm. Highest number of roots was observed on MS medium fortified with 1.0 mg/l NAA (31 roots/shoot), the highest length of roots was relatively more on 1 mg/l IBA (2.96 cm) (Fig. 3g; Table 3).

3.1.6. *Ex vitro* acclimatization and hardening:

The plantlets obtained from *in vitro* culture are delicate and require careful acclimatization to survive outside the controlled environment of the tissue culture lab. In the given study, the plantlets are first transferred to small pots composed of sterilized potting mixture, such as a combination of peat, perlite, and vermiculite (Fig. 3h). These pots are kept in a high humid environment, often under plastic covers or in a misting chamber, to reduce transplant shock. Gradually, the plantlets are exposed to lower humidity and natural light conditions to harden them off. This process can take several weeks, during which the plantlets develop stronger root systems and adapt to the external environment.

Table 2: The effects of KN, BAP, TDZ and NAA combination on multiple shoot induction from shoot bud explants in *Z. zerumbet*.

Hormones (mg/L)	Morphogenic Response	No. of shoots Mean ± SE	Length of shoots Mean ± SE
KN+NAA			
0.2+0.4	S+R	1.33±0.33	7.66±0.33
0.4+0.4	S+R	**2.33±0.33**	**9.33±0.33**
0.6+0.4	S+R	1.66±0.33	6.00±0.57
0.8+0.4	S+R	1.66±0.66	5.66±0.33
1.0+0.4	S+R	1.00±0.00	6.66±0.33
BAP+KN +NAA			
1.0+0.4+0.4	S+R+C	**3.90±0.00** [a]	2.00±0.57
2.0+0.4+0.4	S+R+C	2.66±0.33 [ab]	**2.46±0.33**
3.0+0.4+0.4	S+R+C	3.66±0.33 [ab]	2.33±0.33
4.0+0.4+0.4	S+R+C	3.33±0.33 [ab]	1.66±0.33
5.0+0.4+0.4	S+R+C	2.33±0.33 [b]	2.00±0.00
BAP+TDZ +NAA			
1.0+1.0+0.4	S+R+C	17.66±0.88 [a]	11.66±0.33 [a]
1.0+2.0+0.4	S+R+C	**20.00±0.57** [b]	**13.66±0.67** [ac]
1.0+3.0+0.4	S+R+C	10.66±0.88 [cd]	11.00±1.00 [a]
1.0+4.0+0.4	S+R+C	13.33±1.45 [cd]	9.33±0.33 [ad]
1.0+5.0+0.4	S+R+C	19.00±0.57 [a]	8.66±0.33 [b]

BAP, 6-benzylaminopurine; KN, Kinetin; NAA, 1-naphthaleneacetic acid; TDZ, Thiadiazurone. Every experiment was conducted three times with twenty replicates. The values indicate the average ± standard error. At the 5% level, the Duncan's new multiple range test indicates that there is no significant difference between mean values that have the same letter within columns.

Table 3: Effect of varying concentrations of auxins (IBA and NAA) on induction of multiple roots from elongated shoots of *Z. zerumbet*.

Hormones (mg/L)	**No. of roots Mean ± SE**	**Length of roots Mean ± SE**
	IBA	
0.5	10.66±0.33[a]	1.33±0.33
1.0	**11.66±0.33[b]**	**2.96±0.33**
1.5	9.33±0.33[a]	1.33±0.33
2.0	8.66±0.33[a]	1.66±0.33
2.5	11.00±0.57[a]	2.00±0.57
	NAA	
0.5	22.66±0.88[a]	1.33±0.33
1.0	**31.00±0.57[b]**	**2.73±0.33**
1.5	30.66±0.88[cd]	2.00±0.57
2.0	27.33±1.45[cd]	2.33±0.33
2.5	19.00±0.57[a]	1.00±0.00

IBA, Indole-3-butyric acid; NAA, 1-naphthaleneacetic acid. All the experiments were conducted 3 times with 20 repetitions each. Values show the standard error plus or minus the mean. Mean values within columns that the differently labelled alphabets indicate significant differemce, according to Duncan's new multiple range test at the 5% level.

3.1.7. RAPD molecular markers for genetic stability assessment:

Micropropagation, while efficient in generating large numbers of plantlets, can sometimes induce genetic variations known as somaclonal variations due to the high rates of cell division and the artificial conditions used. These variations may lead to undesirable traits, which could affect the quality, uniformity, and performance of the plantlets in the field. RAPD analysis serves as a reliable tool to detect such variations at the DNA level, ensuring that the *in vitro*regenerants remain genetically similar to the donor plant.

The banding patterns are analyzed for polymorphism. The presence of polymorphic bands (bands that differ among the *in vitro* propagated plantlets and the donor plant) would suggest genetic variation, while monomorphic bands (bands that are identical in all samples) confirm genetic stability.

In the given study, a total of 10 RAPD primers (AM1, AM2, AM3, AM4, AM5, A6, AM7, AM8, AM9, C12) were used and resulted scorable and reproducible amplifications to analyze *in vitro* grown plantlets (Table. 4). Amplification products found were 57 altogether with a mean number of 5.7 bands per primer. There found no polymorphic banding between mother and *in vitro* regenerated plantlets of *Z. zerumbet*. Maximum number of 8 bands was produced by AM1 and AM9 primers in contrast (Fig. 4 & 5), the least number of 1band was observed with A6 primers. The band range was from 40bp to 2000 bp for all primers together.

This study detected no variations among the micropropagated *Z. zerumbet* plantlets which serve as an evidence that the plant's *in-vitro* propagation method is reliable. Plantlets for the study were taken from rhizomatous buds; it confirms the substantially higher genetic stability of rhizome-based micropropagation systems compared to callus-based regeneration systems.

Table: 4 Details of RAPD primers employed for genetic homogeneity assessment in *Z. zerumbet.*

Primer	**Primer sequence (5'-3')**	**Monomorphic bands bands**	**Polymorhic bands**	**Band range**
AM11	CTCTCTCTCTCTCTCTG	8	0	350-2000bp
AM3	GCATGGCAAGCTGCA	7	0	500-2000bp
AM7	CTTCGGCAGCATCTCTTCAT	6	0	50-100bp
C12	GAGGCGTCGC	5	0	40-100bp
AM 2	GGATGGAATAGTCTC	7	0	1500-above
AM 4	GAGAGAGAGAGAGAGAC	5	0	500-1000bp
AM 5	ACACACACACACACACC	6	0	300-1500bp
A6	TGGCCACCTG	1	0	1700 bp
AM8	CAGTGTGGAAGCCGATTATG	4	0	200-700bp
AM9	ATGTGTTGTCTGGCTTGGTA	8	0	400-1000bp

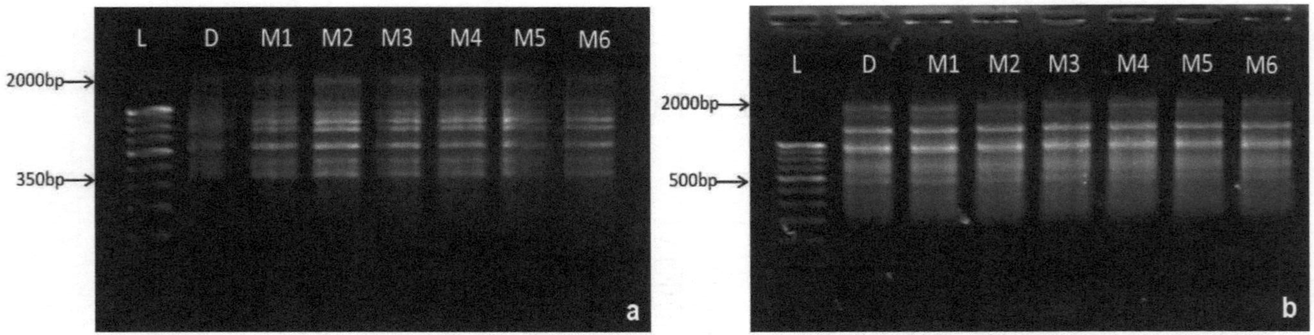

Fig: 4 RAPD banding pattern with primers (a) AM1 and (b) AM3 in both *in vitro* regenerants and field grown donar plant of *Z. zerumbet* (lane 1: ladder, lane 2: donor plant and lane 3-8: micropropagated plants).

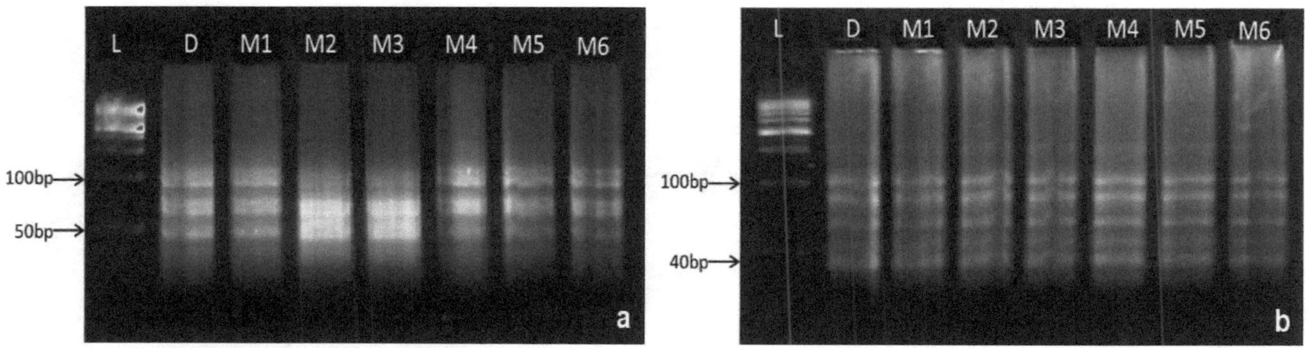

Fig: 5 RAPD banding pattern with primers (a) AM7 and (b) AM12 in both *in vitro* regenerants and field grown donar plant of *Z. zerumbet* (lane 1: ladder, lane 2: donor plant and lane 3-8: micropropagated plants).

3.2. Determination of phytochemical analysis from rhizome extracts of *Z. zerumbet*

3.2.1. Total content of phenolics, flavonoids and tannins:

In the given study, illustrates the content of total phenolics in the rhizome extracts of *Z. zerumbet*. When extracted in ethanolic solvents (48 mg GAE/g DW), *Z. zerumbet* rhizome extract had a greater total polyphenol content than when extracted in other solvents (Fig. 6). The highest quantity was found in the ethanol extract, which was followed by the extracts of acetone, methanol, water, and hexane; similar pattern was observed for the levels of flavonoids (except water exhbiting least) and condensed tannins (Fig. 7 & 8).

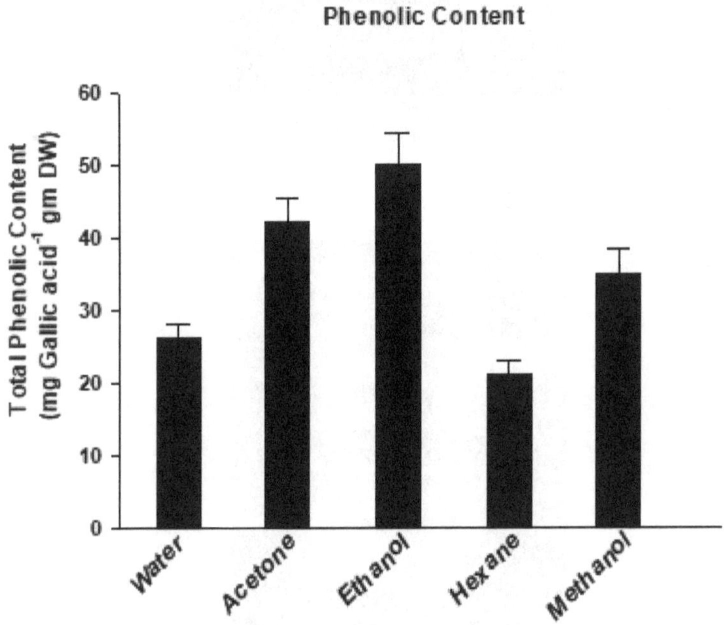

Fig. 6: The total polyphenolics content (expressed as mg gallic acid equivalents^{-1}g dry weight) of *Z. zerumbet* rhizome extracts performed in different solvents.

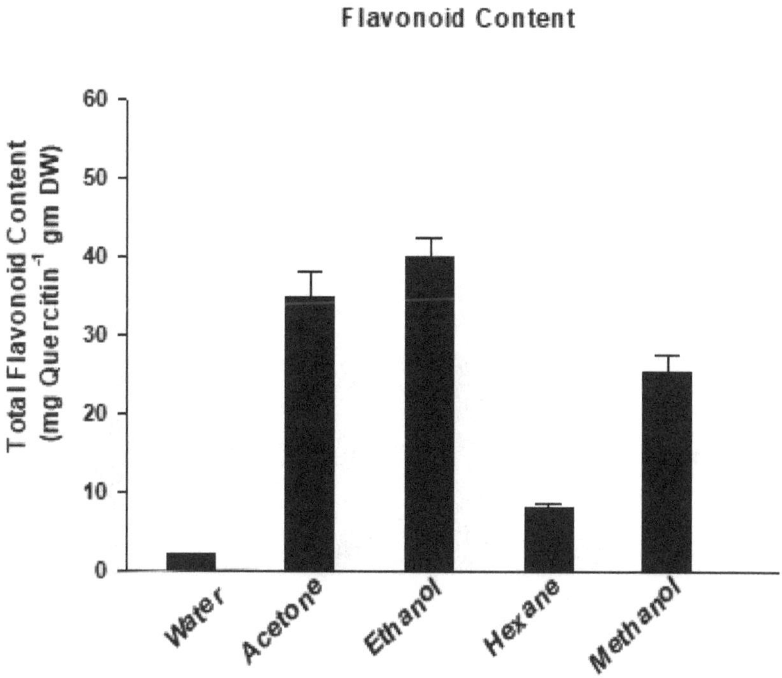

Fig. 7: The total contents of flavonoids (expressed as mg quercitin^{-1} g dry weight) in rhizome extracts of *Z. zerumbet* in different solvents.

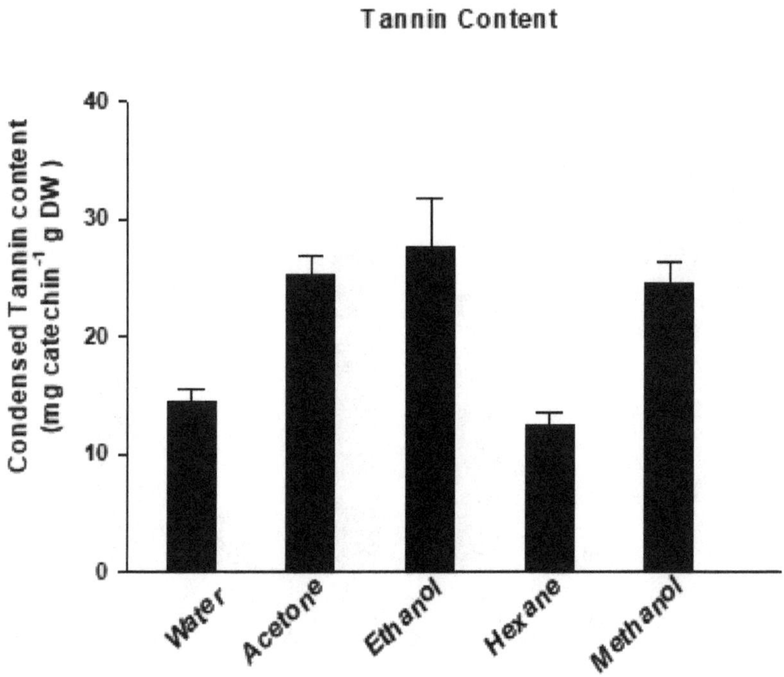

Fig. 8: The total condensed tannin contents (expressed as mg catechin^{-1} g dry weight) in rhizome extracts of *Z. zerumbet* in different solvents.

3.2.2. Total antioxidant capacity:

The capacity of total antioxidants in *Z. zerumbet* rhizome extract varied according to the solvent. Our results depicted that total antioxidant capacity in *Z. zerumbet* rhizome extract was much higher in ethanolic extract, followed by acetone extract, methanol extract, aqueous extract and least was observed in hexane extract (Fig. 9).

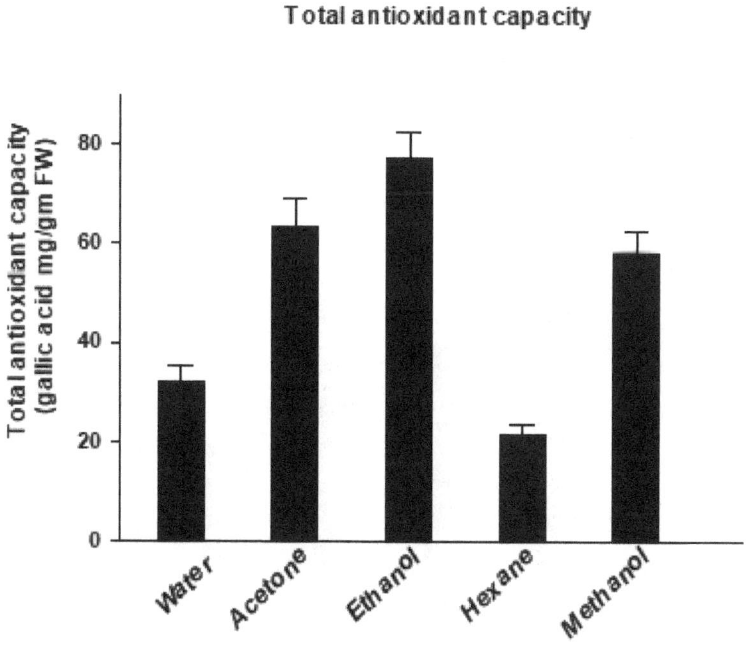

Fig. 9: The capacity of total antioxidants (expressed as mg gallic acid equivalents^{-1} g dry weight) in rhizome extracts of *Z. zerumbet* in different solvents.

3.2.3. Scavenging activity of DPPH radical:

Even the DPPH radical scavenging activity (Fig. 10) exhibited similar pattern as that of total antioxidant capacity. Surprisingly, the rhizome extracts of *Z. zerumbet* extracted in water exhibited significantly high DPPH radical scavenging activity than those collected in other solvents (Fig. 10). Hexane extracts exhibited minimal anti-radical activity and the maximum activity was observed in water followed by ethanol, methanol and acetone.

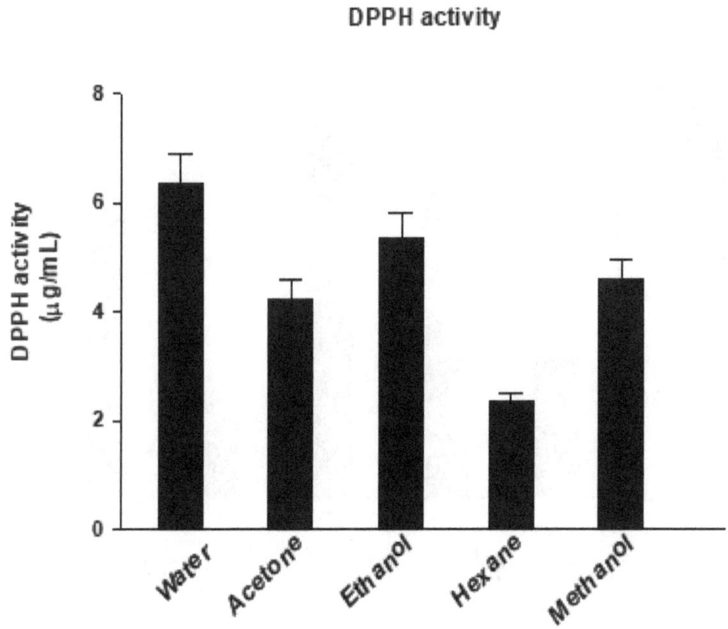

Fig. 10: The scavenging activity of DPPH radical, expressed as median inhibitory concentration (µg/mL), in rhizome extracts of *Z. zerumbet* in different solvents.

3.2.4. Chemical Composition of Extract:

The findings of GC/MS analysis of rhizome extracts of *Z. zerumbet* was presented as Figure 11 highlighting the most important and abundant secondary metabolite compounds such as zerumbone and ginsenol (Table. 5). The secondary metabolites identification was conducted using the NIST library (National Institute of Standards and Technology), which is a comprehensive database of mass spectra. The compounds identified from rhizome extracts were matched against the spectra in the NIST library, ensuring accurate identification. The GC/MS analysis followed standard protocols, which included sample preparation, chromatographic separation, and mass spectrometric detection, to confirm the reliability of the results.

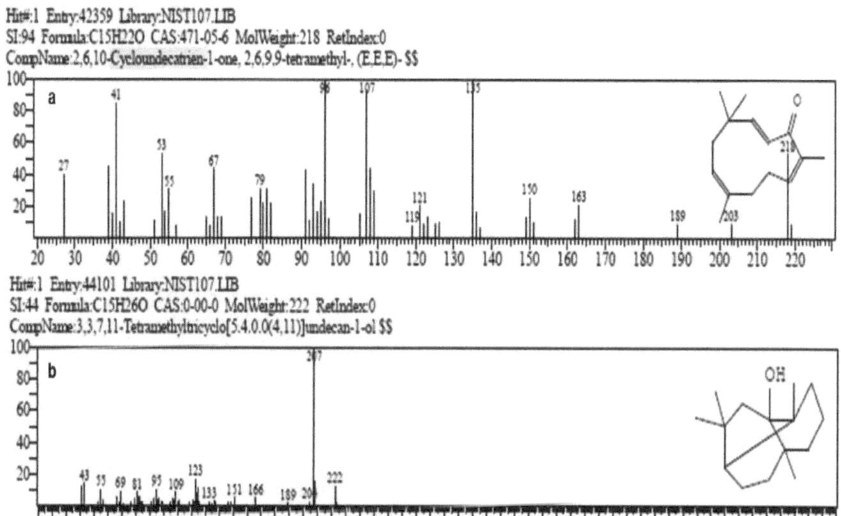

Fig. 11: The GC-MS chromogram of *Z. zerumbet* rhizome methanolic extract with peaks depicting **a)** Zerumbone and **b)** Ginsenol

Table 5 The list of metabolites identified from methanolic extract of *Zingiber zerumbet*

S. No	Compound	Compound type	Mol. wt
1	Zerumbone	Sesquiterpenoid	218
2	Ginsenol	Sesquiterpenoid	222
3	Thymol	Monoterpenoid	222
4	Germacron	Sesquiterpenoid	218
5	Linalool acetate	Monoterpenoid	196
6	Myrtanol	Monoterpenoid	196

3.3. Evaluating the Antibacterial, Antifungal and Insecticidal Activities of *Z. zerumbet* (L.) Roscoe ex Sm Rhizome Extracts

3.3.1. Antibacterial activity:

Zone of inhibition (Fig. 12, Table 6) illustrates that *Z. zerumbet* rhizome extract (500 µg/disc) was efficient against different plant pathogenic bacteria. In contrast to the reference standard kanamycin 30µg/disc, maximum inhibition was obtained against *Xanthomonas spp* (18 mm), *Erwinia spp* (14 mm), and *Pseudomonas syringae* (8 mm) (Table 6). The extract's activity against *Xanthomonas spp.* was demonstrated by the EC50 value of *Z. zerumbet*'s rhizome extracts, which was 156.12 µg mL−1. With an EC50 value of 399.33 µg mL−1, it exhibited considerable action against *Erwinia spp.*, but its EC50 value of 986.17 µg mL−1 indicated negligible control over *Pseudomonas syringae*. Kanamycin (30 µg/disc) showed excellent results against *Xanthomonas spp* (<31 µg mL^{-1}), *Erwinia spp* (<67 µg mL^{-1}) and *Pseudomonas syringae* (<23 µg mL^{-1}).

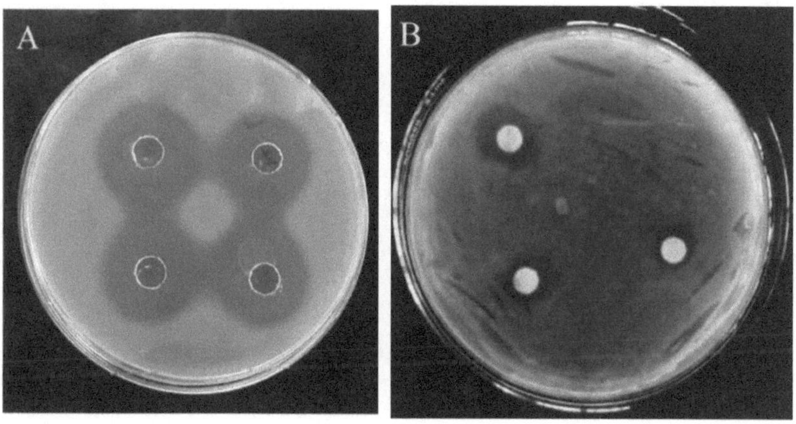

Fig. 12. Inhibitory effect of *Z. zerumbet* rhizome extract on the bacterial growth against tested bacterial pathogen. (A) *Xanthomonas axonopodis pv. Malvacearum* (B) *Erwinia aroideae*

Table 6. Antibacterial activities of the *Z. zerumbet* (L.) rhizome extract.

Test bacterial strains	Zone of Inhibition Diameter (mm)		EC_{50}	
	Extract 500 µg/disc	Std. Kanamycin 30 µg/disc	Extract 500 µg/disc	Std. Kanamycin 30 µg/disc
Xanthomonas spp	18	28	156.12	<31
Erwinia spp	14	25	399.33	<67
Pseudomonas syringae	08	26	986.17	< 23

3.3.2 Antifungal activity:

Data on the fungicidal activity of synthetic drugs carbendazim, which acted as positive control, and *Z. zerumbet* rhizome extracts are shown in Table 7. Our results demonstrated the high inhibition of *Z. zerumbet* rhizome extract (500 μg/disc) against *Rhizoctonia solani* (36 mm), *Fusarium oxysporum* (23 mm) and *Colletotrichum capsici* (11 mm) in comparison to reference standard carbendezim 50 μg/disc (Fig. 13; Table 7). The rhizome extracts of *Z. zerumbet* showed action against *R. solani*, as evidenced by their EC50 value of 164.43 μg mL^{-1}. With an EC50 value of 432.21 μg mL^{-1}, it exhibited moderate activity against *F. oxysporum*, while its EC50 value of 656.23 μg mL^{-1} indicated that it offered the least control over *C. capsici*. Carbendazim showed excellent results against three fungi; *R. solani* (< 22 μg mL^{-1}), *F. oxysporum* (< 34 μg mL^{-1}) and *C. capsici* (< 51 μg mL^{-1}).

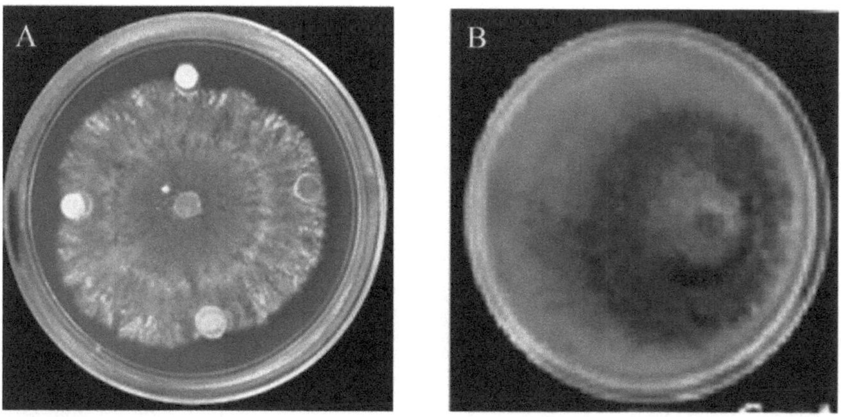

Fig. 13. The *Z. zerumbet* rhizome extract inhibitory effect on the fungal mycelial growth against tested fungal pathogen. (a) *Rhizoctonia solani* (b) *Colletotrichum capsici.*

Table 7. Antifungal activities of the *Z. zerumbet* (L.) rhizome extract.

Fungal strains	Zone of Inhibition Diameter (mm)		EC_{50}	
	Extract 500 µg/disc	Std. Carbendezim 50 µg/disc	Extract 500 µg/disc	Std. Carbendezim 50 µg/disc
Rhizoctonia solani	36	42	164.43	<22
Fusarium oxysporum	23	45	432.21	<34
Colletotrichum capsici	11	46	656.23	< 51

3.3.3. Aphicidal activity:

The data in Table 8 demonstrate the *Z. zerumbet* rhizome extract's aphicidal activity against *A. gossypii*, the cotton aphid. The findings revealed that 87.0% mortality was observed over a 72-hour exposure period at a 500 μg mL−1 concentration (Fig. 14).

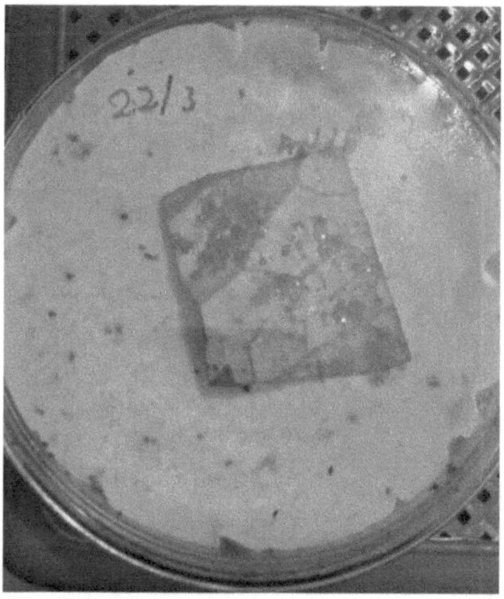

Fig. 14: Mortality studies of *Aphis gossypii* by the addition of 500 mg of *Zingiber zerumbet* rhizome extract

Table 8. Insecticidal activities of the *Zingiber zerumbet* (L.) rhizome extract.

Extract	**Concentration (μg/ml)**	**Insects (no's)**	**Number of insect dead**				**Mortality (%)**
			0 h	**24 h**	**48 h**	**72 h**	
Z. zerumbet rhizome extract	500	15	0	6	9	13	87

4. DISCUSSION

The given study envisaged on the successful establishment *in vitro* regeneration method of *Zingiber zerumbet* and assessment of micro propagated plantlets genetic stability, along with the identification of its potent bioactive compounds. The antimicrobial, antifungal, and insecticidal properties of its rhizome extracts underscore the plant's potential as a valuable resource in developing natural biocides for agricultural use.

4.1.1. Establishment of *in-vitro* regeneration of *Z. zerumbet:*

The given study aimed at establishing *in vitro* propagation of *Zingiber zerumbet* from rhizome bud explants involves a series of carefully controlled steps to ensure successful tissue culture. Initially, our study focused on selecting *Zingiber* zerumbet rhizomes that were disease-free and healthy. To get rid of soil and debris, these rhizome buds are thoroughly cleaned by flowing water from the faucet. The rhizome explants were then thoroughly rinsed with distilled water after being immersed in a detergent solution (e.g., 2-3 drops of Tween 20) for 15-20 minutes. After being soaked in 70% ethanol for one to two minutes, the rhizomes were treated for five to ten minutes with either a solution of 1-2% sodium hypochlorite (NaOCl) or 0.1% (w/v) mercuric chloride ($HgCl_2$) (Fig. 2). To get rid of all traces of the sterilizing agent, the rhizome explants were rinsed 3 to 5 times using sterile distilled water. Every step of the sterilization process was performed in laminar airflow chamber.

During every stage of *Zingiber* zerumbet's *in vitro* propagation, the Murashige and Skoog (MS) medium was prepared freshly (Table 1). To aid in solidification, 0.8% agar and 3% sucrose was added to the MS medium. Plant growth regulators (PGRs) such as BAP and TDZ at doses ranging from 2 to 5 mg/L were used. The medium's pH was brought down to 5.8 prior to autoclaving. The medium was autoclaved at at 121°C, 15 lbs pressure for period of 15-20 min. The explants were inoculated under sterile conditions, by cutting them into small pieces containing the bud (1-2 cm in size). These pieces of explants (bud side up) inoculated on the prepared MS medium under sterile environment performed in laminar flow hood. Seal the culture vessels with parafilm or plastic wrap to prevent contamination. The cultures were incubated in a standard growth conditions at 24-26°C with a 16 h light/8 h dark photoperiod under light intensity of 2000-3000 lux. We monitored the cultures regularly for contamination and growth. Within 2-4 weeks, we observed shoot initiation from the rhizome buds (Fig.2).

After initial shoots are established (2-3 cm), transfer them to fresh MS medium containing a containing 1 mg/L BAP, 2 mg/L TDZ, and 0.4 mg/L NAA for further multiplication (Table 2; Fig. 3). Subculture the shoots every 3-4 weeks to fresh medium to enhance shoot proliferation. The explant produced the more number of shoots, with 20 shoots developing from each explant. This indicates that the explant was highly responsive to the culture conditions, leading to prolific shoot production. Remarkably, about 80% of the shoots that were induced in MS medium enriched with 1 mg/L BAP, 2 mg/L TDZ, and 0.4 mg/L NAA (Table 2; Fig. 3) medium also started to develop roots simultaneously. This is somewhat unusual, as rooting often requires a separate medium with a higher auxin concentration. Table 3 shows that the NAA in the MS medium promoted optimal root growth. Our research's conclusions showed that cytokinins (BAP, TDZ) and auxins (NAA) worked in concert to promote the best possible *in vitro* root formation and elongation of shoots (Table 2). This could be explained by the additional role that cytokines especially TDZ during the plant growth and development, as shown by earlier research (Talla et al. 2019; Talla et al. 2022). When the plantlets had developed a strong root system, they were moved to tiny pots with sterile soil mixture. To help the plantlets become used to their new surroundings, the pots were gradually opened over the course of a week after being covered with plastic to retain humidity. This method should yield healthy *Zingiber zerumbet* plants that are genetically uniform and true to the parent plant.

Similar to our study, several other *in vitro* methods, including direct and indirect regeneration, have been followed for *Z. zerumbet* till now. Finding the most efficient, fastest, and mass multiplicative plant regeneration method for *Z. zerumbet* requires comparison of the validated *in vitro* approaches and their efficacy. One of the key strategies for the growth and multiplication of genetically homogeneous plantlets is direct organogenesis *via* multiple shoot generation (Chavan et al. 2014; Dey et al. 2020; Kshirsagar et al. 2021). Hsu et al. (1991) made the firstly reported direct shoot multiplication for *Z. zerumbet* propagation. After being induced on liquid MS media fortified with 2 mg/l of BAP and 3% sucrose, the shoots were moved to 4.0 mg/l of BAP to facilitate their multiplication (4.78 shoots). The effectiveness of liquid or solid MS media on shoot multiplication was examined by the authors; shoot production was highest with liquid media. Idris et al. (2007) generated *Z. zerumbet* rhizomes using an *in vitro* growth technique and evaluated the secondary metabolites accumulation after a 16-year gap.

As contamination of fungus and bacteria is the major challenge to overcome in tissue culture, there would be a deployment of different disinfectants during sterilization process. It was quite familiar from several studies that mercuric chloride was successfully employed as disinfectant during surface sterilization process (Khaskheli et al. 2022; Permadi et al. 2023). Our results were in corroboration with the findings of Stanly and Keng (2007) with similar simultaneous shoot and root formation in *Z. zerumbet* and several other studies suggested that using a mixed medium reduced the time required for plant regeneration (Talla et al. 2019; Talla et al. 2022). Other *Zingiber*aceae species have reported the role of BAP in shoot proliferation (Al-Taha et al. 2020; George et al. 2022). Auxins are important in inducing shoot buds from a variety of *Zingiber*aceae plants, including *Alpinia galanga* (Sahoo et al. 2020); *Zingiber officinale* (Miri et al. 2020); *Kaempferia kalanga* (Shofiyani et al. 2023); and *Curcuma zedoaria* (Hussain et al. 2023).

Even though there are many advantages to using tissue culture to propagate plants, the plantlets produced from the tissue culture may differ from one another. For this reason, evaluating genetic stability is essential to maintaining the similarity of the plants. In addition to assessing plant diversity and resolving issues with plant identification, molecular markers are essential for verifying the genetic integrity of *in vitro* raised plantlets (Ranemma and Reddy, 2017; Dey et al. 2021; Tikendra et al. 2021; Venkateshgoud and Reddy, 2024). Few studies examined the role of molecular markers in the genetic stability evaluation of *Z. zerumbet*, despite the fact that many papers for the genus *Zingiber* indicated their usefulness for evaluating genetic uniformity.

4.1.2. Assesment of genetic fidelity in micro propagated *Z. zerumbet* plantlets:

In the given study, the RAPD markers were chosen for their ease of application and low cost, as well as their usefulness in detecting variability in DNA sequences across *in vitro* preserved plantlets (Sharim and Shamsiah, 2021; Sarker et al. 2023). Therefore in this study, we utilized 10 different RAPD primers (AM1, AM2, AM3, AM4, AM5, A6, AM7, AM8, AM9, C12) to perform DNA amplification (Table. 4). The amplifications resulting from these primers were scorable and reproducible, meaning the bands produced were clear and consistent across repeated experiments. This reliability is crucial for accurate genetic analysis. Across all 10 primers, a total of 57 distinct DNA bands were observed. On average, each primer produced 5.7 bands. This suggests that the primers were effective in generating multiple DNA fragments, providing a good representation of the genetic material being analyzed. The DNA fragment size (bands) ranged from 40 base pairs (bp) to 2000 bp. This indicates the diversity of the amplified DNA fragments in terms of their lengths, which is typical in RAPD analysis due to the random nature of primer binding. The present study demonstrated no polymorphic bands among the donar plants and the micropropagated plantlets. Polymorphism refers to variations in the DNA sequence that led to different band patterns between samples. The absence of polymorphic bands indicates that the *in vitro* raised plantlets are genetically identical to the donar plants, suggesting that the tissue culture process did not introduce any detectable genetic changes.

In the given study, the primers AM1 and AM9 (Fig. 4 and 5) produced the highest number of bands, with 8 bands each. This suggests that these primers were particularly effective in amplifying multiple regions of the genome in *Zingiber zerumbet.* In contrast, the A6 primer produced only a single band. This indicates that A6 was less effective in amplifying diverse regions of the genome, or it may have a more specific binding site that only amplified a single fragment. The range of band sizes from 40 bp to 2000 bp indicates that the RAPD primers were able to amplify DNA fragments of different sizes, from very short sequences (40 bp) to relatively long ones (2000 bp). This wide range is typical in RAPD analysis and demonstrates the capability of the primers in targeting various regions of the genome. To conclude with that the no polymorphic bands were observed among the donar plants and the *in vitro* plantlets, indicating that the tissue culture process preserved the genetic integrity of the plantlets.

Our results are in corroboration with the reported data, Mohanty et al. (2012) conducted periodic evaluations of the genetic integrity of *Z. zerumbet in vitro* produced clones using RAPD and ISSR analysis, and found that all regenerants exhibited genetic uniformity. Das et al. (2013) used RAPD and ploidy analysis to successfully confirm the cytogenetic integrity of *Z. zerumbet* micropropagated plantlets. The genetic stability of *Z. zerumbet* and other 8 ginger species' *in vitro* rhizome-derived plantlets was evaluated (Mohanty et al. 2014).

4.2. Phytochemistry of Z. zerumbet rhizome extract:

Our study determined the phytochemical composition and biological activity of rhizome extracts from *Zingiber zerumbet.* By analyzing these aspects, the researchers sought to understand the potential applications of the extracts, particularly in terms of their medicinal and pesticidal properties.

The study discusses the analysis of the total phenol content, flavonoid levels and condensed tannins in *Zingiber zerumbet* rhizome extracts when using different solvents. Total phenols are a measure of the polyphenolic compounds and these are quite familiar for their antioxidant properties, and their concentration can indicate the extract's potential bioactivity. The study found that when *Zingiber zerumbet* rhizome was extracted using ethanol, the total phenol content was maximum, with a value of 48 mg GAE/g DW (milligrams of gallic acid equivalents per gram of dry weight). The phenol content in the ethanol extract was considerably high than in extracts made using other solvents such as acetone, methanol, water, and hexane. This indicates that ethanol was appropriate solvent for extraction of polyphenols from *Zingiber zerumbet* rhizomes (Fig. 6).

A class of polyphenolic chemicals termed as flavonoids is well-known for having antibacterial, anti-inflammatory, and antioxidant properties. They are crucial indicators of plant extracts' potential for therapeutic use. The present study found a similar pattern in flavonoid content as observed with total phenols, where ethanol extraction yielded the highest flavonoid levels. Following ethanol, acetone and methanol extracts showed relatively high flavonoid content, while hexane and water extracts had lower levels. Notably, water extracts exhibited the least amount of flavonoids, which is consistent with the lower efficiency of water in extracting non-polar or moderately polar compounds like flavonoids (Fig. 7).

Condensed tannins are a type of polyphenol that influence the antioxidant capacity of the extract. They can also have astringent properties and play roles in plant defense mechanisms. The pattern observed for condensed tannins was similar to that of total phenols and flavonoids. Ethanol was the most effective solvent for extracting condensed tannins from the rhizome, followed by acetone, methanol, hexane, and water. Again, water extracts were less effective, likely due to the mild solubility of tannins in water compared to organic solvents (Fig. 8).

Our findings suggested that ethanol is the best suitable solvent for extraction of phenolic compounds, flavonoids, and tannins from *Zingiber zerumbet* rhizomes, making it the most suitable choice for maximizing the bioactive potential of the extracts. Given the high levels of the biologically active compounds in ethanol extract, it is likely that the ethanol- extracted *Zingiber zerumbet* rhizome would exhibit the strongest biological activity, such as antioxidant and antimicrobial effects.

The study also discusses the variation in *Zingiber zerumbet* rhizome extracts' total antioxidant capacity and DPPH radical scavenging activity dependent on the extraction solvent. The capacity of total antioxidants in *Zingiber zerumbet* rhizome extracts differed depending on the solvent used for extraction. Antioxidant capacity refers to the capability of the extract to neutralize free radicals, thereby preventing oxidative damage. The extract obtained using ethanol had the highest total antioxidant capacity (Fig. 9). This suggests that ethanol was particularly effective at extracting compounds with strong antioxidant properties, such as polyphenols and flavonoids, which to contribute remarkably to antioxidant potential of plant extracts.

Following ethanol, the acetone extract exhibited the next highest antioxidant capacity, although it was slightly lower than that of the ethanol extract (Fig. 9). The methanol extract also demonstrated a good antioxidant capacity, but it was lower than that of both ethanol and acetone extracts. The extract obtained using water showed a lower antioxidant capacity compared to the organic solvents (ethanol, acetone, and methanol). Despite water's ability to extract polar compounds, its effectiveness in extracting antioxidant compounds appeared to be less than that of the organic solvents. The extract obtained using hexane had the lowest total antioxidant capacity. Hexane, being a non-polar solvent, is less effective in extracting polar antioxidant compounds, which likely contributed to the lower antioxidant capacity (Fig. 9).

The rhizome extracts' DPPH radical-scavenging activity and total antioxidant capacity exhibited a comparable pattern. The stable free radical DPPH was frequently employed to assess the antioxidants' capacity to scavenge free radicals in plant extracts. It was quite interesting to note that the aqueous extract had DPPH radical-scavenging activity that was noticeably higher than that of other organic solvents, including methanol and acetone (Fig. 10). Considering that the water extract's overall antioxidant capacity was lower, this was a little surprising. Even though they don't make up as much of the total antioxidant capacity, certain polar antioxidant chemicals that are particularly good at scavenging DPPH radicals may be the cause of the high DPPH activity in the water extract.

Compounds such as certain flavonoids, polyphenols, or other water-soluble antioxidants might be more efficiently extracted in water and exhibit potent radical- scavenging activity (Fig. 10). The ethanol extract also demonstrated strong DPPH radical- scavenging activity, consistent with its high total antioxidant capacity. This reinforces the idea that ethanol effectively extracts a broad range of antioxidant compounds. Both the methanol and acetone extracts showed moderate DPPH activity, which aligns with their performance in the total antioxidant capacity test. These solvents are effective in extracting both polar and non-polar compounds, leading to a balanced antioxidant profile. The hexane solvent extract exhibited the lowest scavenging activity of DPPH radical, consistent with its poor performance in total antioxidant capacity. This further emphasizes that hexane is not an effective solvent for extracting the antioxidant compounds from *Zingiber zerumbet* rhizomes.

The results demonstrate the significant impact polarity of solvent on the antioxidant compounds extraction. As a moderately polar solvent, ethanol effectively extracts a wide range of antioxidant compounds, leading to high total antioxidant capacity and DPPH activity. Despite being highly polar, water's ability to extract specific antioxidant compounds resulted in unexpectedly high DPPH activity, suggesting that certain water-soluble compounds are highly effective at scavenging free radicals. The non-polar nature of hexane makes it less effective in extracting the predominantly polar antioxidant compounds, leading to lower antioxidant activity across both measures.

The presented data was in agreement with previous report in which phenols extracted in various solvents (acetone, dimethyl formamide, ethanol, ethyl acetate, methanol and propanol) (Tan et al. 2012). The extent of polymerization of phenols and its solubility with the extraction solvent, the kind of solvent, the phenols interaction with other plant elements, and the development of insoluble complexes significantly affect the recovery of polyphenols from plant materials (Galvez et al. 2005). The antioxidant activity variations attribute to changes in their polarity of solvents used. Moreover, phenolic solubility is enhanced by solvent polarity (Naczk and Shahidi, 2006). For this reason, defining a consistent protocol for the plant phenols extraction is challenging. The least polar solvents are thought to be appropriate for lipophilic phenols extraction, while polar solvents are employed for extraction of phenols with hydrophilic nature (Alothman et al. 2009).

Gas chromatography-Mass spectrometry (GC-MS) is an advanced analytical technique used to quantify and identify the chemical components of the sample. In the given study, GC-MS was employed to separate and identify the individual compounds in the *Zingiber zerumbet* rhizome extracts (Fig. 11 and Table. 5). The analysis revealed a high presence of sesquiterpenes, specifically ginsenol and zerumbone (Fig. 11). Ginsenol, sesquiterpene is known for its anti-inflammatory and potentially anti-cancer properties.

Zerumbone, a well-known bioactive compound in *Zingiber zerumbet*, zerumbone was extensively studied for its anticancer, anti-inflammatory, antimicrobial and antioxidant activities. Idris et al. (2007) investigated that the zerumbone accumulation with 40.25% and 9 other metabolites were confirmed by GC-MS profiling of *Z. zerumbet* rhizomes. These metabolites include cis-α-bisabolene; camphene; 3,7-cyclodecadien-1- one; 2,10-dimethyl-3-(1-met) curdione; 1H-purine-2,6-dione-theobromine; 3,7-cyclodecadiene-germacrone; α-humulene; β-selinene and (Z)-2,3,dihydro-1H-cyclonona zerumbone (Shinija et al. 2009).

Research on the rhizome of *Z. zerumbet* has been demonstrated to vary in composition depending on the country, India (Rawat et al. 2024), Malaysia (Preshahdin et al. 2023), and Bangladesh (Aunjum et al. 2020). Because of its high zerumbone content from India, rhizomes oil was also discovered to have fungicidal activity against phytopathogenic fungi, including *Rhizoctonia solani, Sclerotium rolfsii, and Macrophomina phaseolina* (Rana et al. 2017). Hence, in the further study we focused on biocidal activity of *Z. zerumbet* on different plant pathogenic bacteria, fungi and insect pest.

4.3. Biocidal activities of *Z. zerumbet* rhizome extracts:

The study investigates the antibacterial, antifungal and pesticidal activity of *Zingiber zerumbet* rhizome extracts against various plant pathogenic organisms by analyzing the zone of inhibition and EC50 values.

4.3.1. Antibiotic Activity Evaluation

The *Zingiber zerumbet* rhizome extract was tested at a concentration of 500 µg/disc against different plant pathogenic bacteria. The zone of inhibition refers to the area around a disc where fungal growth is prevented, indicating the efficacy of the extract in inhibiting the pathogen. The extract showed the maximum inhibition against *Xanthomonas axonopodis* pv. *Malvacearum*, with 18 mm zone of inhibition (Fig. 12, Table 6). This suggests that the extract is particularly effective against this pathogen. The extract also demonstrated significant inhibition against *Erwinia aroideae*, at zone of inhibition (14 mm). This indicates a moderate level of antifungal activity. The extract showed some inhibitory effect against *Pseudomonas syringae*, with small zone of inhibition (8 mm), suggesting relatively lower efficacy against this pathogen compared to the others (Fig. 12; Table 6). Kanamycin (30 µg/disc), a standard antibiotic used as a reference in the study, was highly effective against all three pathogens, indicating its broad-spectrum activity.

EC50 (half maximal effective concentration) is the concentration of extract needed to inhibit 50% of the pathogen's growth. Lower EC50 values indicate higher efficacy of the extract. The rhizome extract had an EC50 value of 156.12 µg/mL against *Xanthomonas axonopodis* pv. Malvacearum. This relatively low value suggests that the extract is quite potent against this pathogen, though not as potent as kanamycin, which had an EC50 of less than 31 µg/mL. The extract's EC50 value against *Erwinia aroideae* was 399.33 µg/mL, indicating moderate effectiveness. In comparison, kanamycin had a much lower EC50 value of less than 67 µg/mL, demonstrating its superior efficacy. The rhizome extract showed minimal control over *Pseudomonas syringae*, with an EC50 value of 986.17 µg/mL, indicating weak activity (Fig. 12; Table 6). Kanamycin, on the other hand, had a much lower EC50 value of less than 23 µg/mL, showing its strong effectiveness.

The *Zingiber zerumbet* rhizome extract exhibited strong antibacterial activity against *Xanthomonas axonopodis* pv. *Malvacearum* and moderate activity against *Erwinia aroideae*. However, its effectiveness against *Pseudomonas syringae* was limited, as indicated by the small zone of inhibition and high EC50 value. While the extract is not as potent as kanamycin, it could still be considered as a natural alternative or complement to synthetic antibiotics, particularly for pathogens like *Xanthomonas axonopodis* pv. *Malvacearum*. The moderate and lower effectiveness against *Erwinia aroideae* and *Pseudomonas syringae*, respectively, suggests that further refinement or combination with other extracts or treatments might be necessary to improve efficacy (Fig. 12; Table 6). The study highlights the potential of *Zingiber zerumbet* rhizome extract as a natural antibiotic, particularly against specific plant pathogens like *Xanthomonas axonopodis* pv. *Malvacearum*. This could offer a more sustainable and ecofriendly alternative to synthetic antibiotic. The varying levels of effectiveness against different pathogens suggest that the extract might be best used in targeted applications, rather than as a broad-spectrum antibiotic.

Our findings are in line with the study which illustrated that *Z. zerumbet* extract exhibited potent antibiotic and fungicidal activity (Kader et al. 2011). This study highlighted the presence of phytochemicals with antibacterial and antifungal property in ethanolic extract of *Z. zerumbet*. The *Z. zerumbet* rhizome extract was also possessed abundant polyphenolic compounds, which contribute to its antioxidant properties. These findings suggest that *Z. zerumbet* rhizome extract may have promising antibacterial properties against plant pathogenic bacteria. Further research is warranted to explore its full potential and understand the mechanism of action.

4.3.2. Antifungal Activity Evaluation

The study explores the fungicidal activity of *Zingiber zerumbet* rhizome extracts and compares it with a synthetic fungicide, carbendazim, which is used as a positive control. The data from (Fig. 13; Table 7) highlights the varying levels of effectiveness of the rhizome extract against different fungal pathogens. The *Zingiber zerumbet* rhizome extract was tested at a dosage of 500 μg/disc. The zone of inhibition is a measure of the extract's potential to inhibit fungal growth around the disc. Larger zones indicate higher fungicidal activity, the rhizome extract showed the maximum inhibition against *Rhizoctonia solani*, with a zone of inhibition measuring 36 mm (Fig. 13; Table 7). This indicates strong antifungal activity against this particular pathogen. The extract also demonstrated significant activity against *Fusarium oxysporum*, producing zone of inhibition (23 mm), reflecting moderate effectiveness. The extract had a relatively smaller inhibitory effect on *Colletotrichum capsici*, with zone of inhibition (11 mm), indicating that its effectiveness against this fungus is lower compared to the other two (Fig. 13; Table 7).

Carbendazim (30 μg/disc), a widely used synthetic fungicide, served as the positive control to benchmark the effectiveness of the rhizome extract. Carbendazim exhibited a very strong inhibitory effect on *Rhizoctonia solani*, with a much lower EC50 value of less than 22 μg/mL, indicating its superior fungicidal activity. Against *Fusarium oxysporum*, carbendazim also showed strong efficacy with an EC50 value of less than 34 μg/mL, significantly better than the rhizome extract. Carbendazim was most effective against *Colletotrichum capsici*, with an EC50 value of less than 51 μg/mL (Fig. 12; Table 7), demonstrating its strong fungicidal action across all tested pathogens. The EC50 value is the concentration required to inhibit the fungal growth by 50%. Lower EC50 values indicate higher fungicidal efficacy. The rhizome extract had an EC50 value of 164.43 μg/mL against *Rhizoctonia solani*. Although this value is higher than that of carbendazim, it still reflects strong activity, particularly for a natural extract. The extract's EC50 value against *Fusarium oxysporum* was
432.21 μg/mL, indicating moderate fungicidal activity. This is significantly less effective than carbendazim, but still noteworthy for a natural product (Fig. 13; Table 7). The extract showed the least effectiveness against *Colletotrichum capsici*, with an EC50 value of 656.23 μg/mL, reflecting low activity compared to the other pathogens. Carbendazim's much lower EC50 value indicates its strong efficacy against this fungus.

The *Zingiber zerumbet* rhizome extract demonstrated the most substantial fungicidal activity against *Rhizoctonia solani*, followed by moderate activity against *Fusarium oxysporum*, and the least activity against *Colletotrichum capsici*. The high EC50 values for *Fusarium oxysporum* and *Colletotrichum capsici* suggest that higher concentrations of the extract would be required for effective control. While the rhizome extract shows promise, it is less effective than carbendazim, especially for *Colletotrichum capsici*. The lower EC50 values of carbendazim across all pathogens highlight its superior efficacy as a synthetic fungicide. However, the natural extract's performance, particularly against *Rhizoctonia solani*, suggests it could be a viable alternative or complement in integrated pest management strategies.

Research has shown that *Zingiber sp* rhizome extract possesses anti-fungal properties against various fungi (Xi et al. 2022). In studies conducted at a dosage of 400 µg/disc, the extract displayed mild to moderate activity of antibiotic and fungicidal action, as evidenced by the 6 mm to 10 mm diameter zone of inhibition. These findings suggest that *Zingiber* rhizome extract has the potential to restrict the growth of fungal pathogens.

The study clearly illustrates that *Zingiber zerumbet* rhizome extract has the capability to develop into a natural fungicide, especially against pathogens like *Rhizoctonia solani*. Its use could reduce reliance on synthetic chemicals, contributing to more sustainable agricultural practices. The extract's varying effectiveness against different fungi suggests that it may be best utilized in specific contexts rather than as a broad-spectrum fungicide. It could be particularly useful in organic farming systems where the usage of synthetic chemicals is restricted. To enhance the extract's efficacy, further research could explore optimizing extraction methods, combining it with other natural or synthetic agents, or increasing its concentration for improved control of less susceptible pathogens like *Fusarium oxysporum* and *Colletotrichum capsici*.

4.3.3. Aphicidal Activity Evaluation

The study evaluates the aphicidal (insect-killing) activity of *Zingiber zerumbet* rhizome extracts against the cotton aphid, *Aphis gossypii*, by observing the mortality rate after exposure. The data in Table 8 highlight the effectiveness of the extract in controlling aphid populations. The rhizome extract was tested at a dosage of 500 µg/mL, with aphid mortality assessed after 72 hours of exposure resulting in an 87.0% mortality rate of the cotton aphid, *Aphis gossypii*. This high mortality rate suggests that the extract is highly effective in killing aphids when applied at this concentration (Fig. 14; Table 8). The 72-hour exposure period is significant as it demonstrates the time-dependent effectiveness of the extract (Fig. 14; Table 8). In pest management, understanding the time required to achieve maximum mortality is crucial for optimizing application schedules. An 87.0% mortality rate over this period indicates that the extract has a strong potential to significantly reduce aphid populations in cotton crops. This could lead to reduced damage from aphid infestations, which are known to cause considerable economic losses in agriculture.

While the study focuses on the natural extract, it is common practice to compare such results with those of synthetic aphicides. Although specific data from synthetic controls are not provided in this instance, the high mortality rate achieved by the rhizome extract suggests it could be a viable alternative or supplement to synthetic aphicides. The use of natural extracts like that of *Zingiber zerumbet* is often preferred in integrated pest management (IPM) strategies to reduce the environmental impact caused by synthetic chemicals. The high efficacy observed here supports the extract's potential role in sustainable agriculture. The effectiveness of the *Zingiber zerumbet* rhizome extract likely stems from its bioactive compounds, such as sesquiterpenes and phenolics, which have been previously noted for their insecticidal properties. These compounds may disrupt the nervous system of aphids, inhibit feeding, or cause dehydration, leading to mortality. Understanding the specific mechanisms by which the extract causes aphid mortality could help in refining its application and improving its effectiveness. Further research into isolating and testing these bioactive compounds could lead to the development of more targeted and potent aphicidal agents.

Cotton aphids are a significant pest in cotton production, and controlling their populations is vital to preventing yield losses. The study's results suggest that *Zingiber zerumbet* rhizome extract could be an effective tool in managing aphid infestations, potentially reducing the need for synthetic pesticides and lowering the risk of pesticide resistance. The high mortality rate observed with the natural extract supports its integration into IPM programs. By combining it with other biological and cultural control methods, farmers could achieve more sustainable and effective pest management. The promising results may also encourage the commercial development of *Zingiber zerumbet*-based aphicides. Such products could cater to the growing demand for organic and eco-friendly pest control solutions.

Alternative strategy for minimizing the over exploitation of synthetic pesticides is to employ plants as botanical insecticides (Divekar, 2023). Bioactive substances such terpenoids, alkaloids, flavonoids, steroids and tannins are commonly found in plants that function as bioinsecticides (Miranti and Fatiqin, 2018). It has been shown that a number of plant families contain bioactive chemicals that have insecticidal effects (Fowsiya and Madhumitha, 2020). It has been claimed that members of the *Zingiber*aceae family, and specifically the ginger plant (*Zingiber officinale* R.), have insecticidal qualities (Siregar et al. 2024). In general, plants are prone to attacked by insects, microbes, and mammals typically develop self-defense mechanisms through the production of a range of secondary metabolites, including alkaloids, aromatic compounds, steroids and terpenoids which are likely repulsive or even poisonous to the adversary (Divekar et al. 2022).

It was quite familiar that, *Z. zerumbet* plant has been the subject of prior phytochemical studies that have identified flavonoids, steroids, triterpenoids and alkaloids. It is possible that the presence of these kinds of phyto-constituents is what causes the extract of *Z. zerumbet* rhizome to exhibit insecticidal activity. Drug resistance in phyto-pathogens can significantly reduce the efficacy of certain pesticides (Shcherbakova, 2019). In the given study, we evaluated the biocidal properties of *Z. zerumbet* rhizome extracts on different plant pathogenic bacteria, fungi and insect pests. Our results were in agreement with the reported data and can be helpful in development of *Z. zerumbet* as an alternative biocide against various plant pathogens.

5. SUMMARY AND CONCLUSION

Zingiber zerumbet, also termed as bitter ginger, a perennial plant belong to *Zingiber*aceae family. The *Zingiber zerumbet* rhizomes are enriched with essential oils and various bioactive compounds, such as zerumbone, which has been comprehensively studied for its potential medicinal properties. Traditionally, the rhizomes have been used in various ethnicities for medicinal purposes, including treatments for digestive issues, inflammation, and infections. In recent years, *Zingiber zerumbet* has garnered scientific interest due to potential therapeutic applications. Studies have envisaged on its anti-inflammatory, antimicrobial, antioxidant, and anticancer properties, highlighting its promising role as a natural compounds for pharmaceutical and nutraceutical development. Beyond its medicinal uses, *Zingiber zerumbet al.*so holds potential in agriculture as a natural pesticide, contributing to sustainable farming practices. Overall, *Zingiber zerumbet* is a plant of significant ecological, cultural, and economic value, with a growing body of research supporting its diverse applications in traditional medicine, modern pharmacology, and sustainable agriculture.

5.1. *In vitro* regeneration method from rhizome explants of *Zingiber zerumbet.*

The establishment of *Zingiber* zerumbet *in vitro* culture and the evaluation of genetic integrity were the main objectives of the study. In this study, we used rhizome explants to successfully create an effective and repeatable *in vitro* plant regeneration strategy for *Zingiber* zerumbet Smith. When cultivated on a medium enriched with 1 mg/L BAP, 2 mg/L TDZ, and 0.4 mg/L NAA, the shoot bud explants obtained from rhizomes produced the more number of shoots (20 shoots per explant). Surprisingly, over 80% of the induced rooting occurred on the root induction medium, which was MS media enriched with 1.0 mg/L NAA. Following their acclimatization in a greenhouse, these regenerating plantlets demonstrated a remarkable survival rate of 90%.

5.2. Genetic fidelity assesment of *in vitro* regenerated plantlets of *Z. zerumbet* using RAPD molecular markers

Further, we focused on evaluating the genetic stability of *Zingiber zerumbet* plantlets that were propagated *in vitro* through tissue culture methods. Morphological observations indicated that these micropropagated plantlets appeared similar to the mother plants, suggesting that they maintained their external characteristics. However, to validate the genetic fidelity of these plantlets, Random Amplified Polymorphic DNA (RAPD) molecular markers were employed. In this investigation, a total of 10 RAPD primers, designated as AM1 through AM9 and C12, were utilized to amplify DNA from the *in vitro*-grown plantlets. These primers successfully generated scorable and reproducible amplification patterns, which were then analyzed to compare the genetic makeup of the micro propagated plantlets with that of the mother plants. The RAPD analysis resulted in a total of 57 distinct amplification products, with an mean number of 5.7 bands produced per primer. Notably, primers AM1 and AM9 generated the maximum number of bands (8 each), while the A6 primer produced the fewest, with only one band. The amplified bands size ranged from 40 base pairs (bp) to 2000 bp across all primers. Importantly, no polymorphic bands differences in the DNA profiles were detected between the donor plant and the *in vitro* raised plantlets. This absence of polymorphism indicates that the genetic material of the micro propagated plantlets was identical to that of the donor plant, verifying their genetic uniformity. Our study's findings were significant and the molecular analysis revealed that the genetic profiles of all *in vitro* regenerants were similar to those of the donor plant. This genetic uniformity indicates that the *in vitro* regeneration process not only preserved the physical traits but also maintained the genetic integrity of *Z. zerumbet.*

5.3. Investigation of the phytochemical analysis of *Z. zerumbet* rhizome extracts:

The purpose of the present study was also to gain insight into the biological activities and chemical makeup of *Zingiber zerumbet* rhizome extracts. We focused to examine how the different extraction solvents changed the extract's overall polyphenol concentration and related biological activity. The present study revealed that the total polyphenol content of the extract was considerably higher when the rhizomes were extracted using ethanolic solvents. In particular, 48 mg of gallic acid equivalents (GAE) / gram of dry weight (DW) was used to assess the concentration. The chemicals recognized for their antioxidant qualities, phenols, flavonoids, and tannins, were among the polyphenols that were quantified. The ethanol-derived extract exhibited enhanced antioxidant activity, as demonstrated by capability in scavenging free radicals of DPPH. This indicates that ethanol was highly effective than other solvents in extracting bioactive compounds possessing antioxidant properties from the *Zingiber zerumbet* rhizomes.

To understand the phytochemical status of extract, we deployed gas chromatography - mass spectrometry (GC-MS), a powerful technique for chemical constituents identification and quantification. The analysis revealed that the extract was particularly rich in sesquiterpenes, a class of naturally occurring terpenes with known therapeutic properties. Among these, two compounds stood out: Zerumbone; a major sesquiterpene in the extract, known for its anti-inflammatory, anticancer, and antimicrobial activities. Ginsenol; another significant sesquiterpene, contributing to the bioactivity of the extract.

5.4. Investigation of the antagonistic effect of *Z. zerumbet* rhizome extracts on plant pathogenic bacteria, fungi and insect pest:

Owing to its phytochemical efficiency of *Z. zerumbet*, we aimed at evaluation of antibacterial, antifungal, and pesticidal properties of rhizome extracts from *Zingiber zerumbet*, focusing on their effectiveness against specific pathogens and pests. The rhizome extract was tested against three bacterial pathogens: *Xanthomonas spp.*, *Erwinia spp.*, and *Pseudomonas syringae*. These bacteria are known to cause significant diseases in plants, leading to substantial agricultural losses. The extract exhibited strong antibacterial properties against all tested bacteria, with the most pronounced activity observed against *Xanthomonas spp.* This suggests that the extract could potentially be used as a natural antibacterial agent to manage bacterial infections in plants, especially those caused by *Xanthomonas spp.* The antifungal efficacy of the rhizome extract was assessed against three fungal pathogens: *Rhizoctonia solani*, *Fusarium oxysporum*, and *Colletotrichum capsici*. These fungi are notorious for causing diseases like root rot, wilt, and anthracnose in various crops. The extract demonstrated significant antifungal activity across all tested fungi, with the highest inhibitory effect observed against *Rhizoctonia solani*. This indicates that *Z. zerumbet* rhizome extract could be a potent natural fungicide, particularly effective in control of disease caused by *R. solani*.

Apart from antibiotic and fungicidal properties, the study also explored the pesticidal potential of the extract against the cotton aphid, *Aphis gossypii*, a common pest that infests a wide range of crops. The results were compelling, showing that the rhizome extract caused 87.0% mortality in *A. gossypii* after 72 hours of exposure. This high level of pesticidal activity suggests that the extract could be developed into an effective, natural pesticide for controlling aphid populations in agricultural settings.

Conclusions:

The tissue culture study concludes the successful standardization of an efficient, reliable and reproducible *in vitro* propagation protocol for *Zingiber zerumbet* using rhizome explants. The optimized protocol led to the generation of 20 shoots per explant on 1 mg/L BAP, 2 mg/L TDZ, and 0.4 mg/L NAA, with high rooting efficiency (80%) on MS medium fortified with 1.0 mg/L NAA. The regenerated plantlets are identical to mother plants demonstrated a robust survival rate of 90% when acclimatized under greenhouse conditions. This protocol not only facilitates the mass propagation of *Zingiber zerumbet* but also ensures a reliable method for conservation and commercial cultivation of this valuable species.

The outcome of genetic fidelity study using RAPD molecular markers is crucial because it confirms that the propagation method does not introduce unwanted genetic variations, which could affect the plant's desirable traits. Therefore, this *in vitro* regeneration procedure holds promise as a valuable method for the genetic improvement and conservation of *Zingiber zerumbet*. It ensures the consistent production of genetically stable plantlets, which is essential for both large-scale cultivation and any potential biotechnological applications.

The phytochemical study focused on quantitative by means of photometric methods and qualitative analysis by GC-MS of *Z. zerumbet* rhizome extracts. Our findings conclude that the choice of ethanol as the solvent for extraction maximized the yield of bioactive compounds, particularly polyphenols and sesquiterpenes, from *Zingiber zerumbet* rhizomes. This extract not only showed high antioxidant activity but also contained significant amounts of zerumbone and ginsenol, which could be responsible for its therapeutic potential. The study highlights the importance of solvent selection for extraction process, as it directly influences the phytochemical constituents and biological efficacy of the plant extracts.

The biocidal property evaluation study concluded the broad-spectrum bioactivity of *Zingiber zerumbet* rhizome extract. It demonstrated significant antibacterial effects, particularly against *Xanthomonas spp.*, and strong antifungal action, especially against *Rhizoctonia solani*. Furthermore, the extract showed remarkable pesticidal efficacy, with high mortality rates observed in *Aphis gossypii*. These findings suggest that *Z. zerumbet* rhizome extract could serve as a valuable natural agent in integrated pest and disease management strategies, offering an eco-friendly alternative to synthetic chemicals in agriculture.

REFERENCES

Abdel Wahab SI, Bustamam A, Abdul, Alzubairi AS, Elhassan MM, Mohan S (2009) *In vitro* ultramorphological assessment of apoptosis induced by Zerumbone on (HeLa). *J Biomed Biotechnol* ArticleID 769568, 10 pp

Abdelwahab, SI., Abdul, AB., Zain, ZNM., & Hadi, AHA. (2012). Zerumbone inhibits interleukin-6 and induces apoptosis and cell cycle arrest in ovarian and cervical cancer cells. *International immunopharmacology*, *12*(4), 594-602.

Abdul AB, Adel SA, Nirmala DT, Siddig SI, Zetty ZN, Sharin R *et al.* (2008) Anticancer activity natural compound (zerumbone) extracted from *Zingiber zerumbet* in human HeLa cervical cancer cells. Int J Pharmacol 4:160–168

ALFahdawi, S. M., & Joudah, M. T. (2020). Study On Antibacterial And Antifungal Activity Of Ginger (*Zingiber* officinale) On Selected Pathogenic Microorganism. *Biochemical and Cellular Archives*, *20*(2), 4629-4633.

Alothman, M., Rajeev, A., Karim, A. (2009) Antioxidant capacity andphenolic content of selected tropical fruits from Malaysia, extracted with different solvents, Food Chem. 115 785–788.

Al-Saffar FJ, Ganabadi S, Fakurazi S, Yaakub H, Lip M (2010) Chondroprotective effect zerumboneiodo acetate induced osteoarthritis in rats. J Appl Sci 10(4):248–260

Al-Taha, Huda A., Abdulelah A. Al-Mayah, and Widad A. Abd Al-Behadili. "Efficient *in vitro* regeneration of *Zingiber* officinale Rosc. var. White through shoot tips culture." *Plant Archives* 20, no. 1 (2020): 434-437.

Al-zubairi AS, Abdul AB, Siddig IA, Somchit MN (2007) Genetoxicity of zerumbone in peripheral blood lymphocytes evaluated by cytotoxic test. In: Proceedings of 6th international traditional/complementary medicine conference (INTRACOM'07), PWTC, KualaLumpur, Malaysia

Amarowicz, R., Pegg, R.B., Rahimi, M., Barl, B., Weil, J.A. Free-radical scavenging capacity and antioxidant activity of selected plant species from the Canadian prairies, Food Chem. 84 (2004)551–562.

Andreo, D., & Jorge, N. (2011). Antioxidant capacity and oxidative stability of *Gingiber officinale*

Anis M, Ahmad N. 2016. Plant tissue culture: propagation, conservation and crop improvement. Singapore: Springer, pp 15-44.

Aswati Nair R, Kiran AG, Sivakumar KC, Thomas G (2010) Molecular characterization of an oomycete-responsive PR5 protein gene from *Zingiber zerumbet*. Plant Mol Biol Rep 28:128–135

Aunjum, A., Biswas, R., Nurunnabi, T.R., Rahman, S.M., Billah, M.M., Islam, M.E. and Islam, K.M.D., 2020. Antioxidant and antibacterial activity of three herbs belonging to *Zingiber* genus of Bangladesh. *Advances in Traditional Medicine*, *20*, pp.343-350.

Azizi, A. (2010). Genetic, chemical and agro-morphological evaluation of the medicinal plant Origanum vulgare L. for marker assisted improvement of pharmaceutical quality.

Babar PS, Deshmukh AV, Salunkhe SS, Chavan JJ (2020) Micropropagation, polyphenol content and biological properties of sweet flag (*Acorus calamus*): a potent medicinal and aromatic herb. Vegetos 33:296–303

Baby, S., Dan, M., Thaha, A.R.M., Johnson, A.J., Kurup, R., Balakrishnapillai, P., Lim, C.K., 2009. High content of zerumbone in volatile oils of *Zingiber zerumbet* from southern India and Malaysia. Flavour Fragr. J. 24, 301–308.

Bandara, K.N.P., Kumar, V., Saxena, R.C. and Ramdas, P.K., 2005. Bruchid (Coleoptera: Bruchidae) ovicidal phenylbutanoid from *Zingiber* purpureum. *Journal of economic entomology*, *98*(4), pp.1163-1169.

Bauer AW, Kirby WM, Sherris JC,Turck M.1996. Antibiotic susceptibility testing by standardized single disc method. *Am J Clin Pathol* 44, 493-496

Bensch S, Akesson M (2005) Ten years of AFLP in ecology and evolution: why so few animals? Mol Ecol 14:2899–2914

Bidabadi, S. S., & Jain, S. M. (2020). Cellular, molecular, and physiological aspects of *in vitro* plant regeneration. *Plants*, *9*(6), 702.

Bilal, T., Mushtaq, T., Ahmad, P.I., Gangoo, S.A., Behar, B., Ayoob, B., Farooq, S. and Mushtaq, I., 2022. Botanicals their use as antimicrobial, antifungal and anti insecticides. *The Pharma Innovation. SP-11 (5)*, pp.1521-1528.

Bokyung S, Sonia J, Kwang SA, Yoichi M, Tingfang Y, Sushovan G, Mingyao L, Bhara BB (2008) Zerumbone downregulates chemokine receptor CXCR4 expression leading to inhibition of CXCL12-induced invasion of breast and pancreatic tumor cells. Cancer Res 68:21

Bordia A, Verma SK, Srivastava KC (1997) Effect of ginger (*Zingiber* officinale Rosc) and fenugreek (Trigomella foenumgraecum L.) on blood lipids, blood sugar and platelet aggregation in patients with coronary artery disease. Prostaglandins Leukot Essent Fatty Acids 56:379–384

Boulogne I, Petit P, Ozier-Lafontaine H, Desfontaines L, Loranger-Merciris G (2012) Insecticidal and antifungal chemicals produced by plants: a review. Environ Chem Lett 10:325–347.

Bousquet Y.1990. Beetles associated with stored products in Canada. Canadian Government Publishing Centre. Ottawa 189-192 pp.

Bustamam A, Siddig I, Al-Zubairi AS, Manal MET, Syam MM (2008) Zerumbone: a natural compound with anti-cholinesterase activity. Am J Pharmacol Toxicol 3(3):209–211

Chakraborty, A., Santra, I., Haque, S. M., & Ghosh, B. (2023). *In vitro* conservation of commercial and threatened members of *Zingiber*aceae: an Indian scenario. *Biodiversity and Conservation*, *32*(7), 2155-2195.

Chan, J. S. W., Lim, X. Y., Japri, N., Ahmad, I. F., & Tan, T. Y. C. (2023). *Zingiber zerumbet*: a scoping review of its medicinal properties. *Planta Medica*.

Chan, J. S. W., Lim, X. Y., Japri, N., Ahmad, I. F., & Tan, T. Y. C. (2023). *Zingiber zerumbet*: a scoping review of its medicinal properties. *Planta Medica*.

Chane-Ming, J., Vera, R. and Chalchat, J.C., 2003. Chemical composition of the essential oil from rhizomes, leaves and flowers of *Zingiber zerumbet* Smith from Reunion Island. *Journal of Essential Oil Research*, *15*(3), pp.202-205.

Chaungab HC, Chi-Tang H, Tzou-Chi H (2008) Anti-hypersensitive and anti-inflammatory activities of water extract of *Zingiber zerumbet* (L.). Food Agric Immunol 19(2): 117–129

Chavan JJ, Gaikwad NB, Dixit GB, Yadav SR, Bapat VA (2018) Biotechnological interventions for propagation, conservation and improvement of 'lantern flowers' (*Ceropegia* spp.). S Afr J Bot 114:192–216

Chavan JJ, Gaikwad NB, Umdale SD, Kshirsagar PR, Bhat KV, Yadav SR (2014) Efficiency of direct and indirect shoot organogenesis, molecular profiling, secondary metabolite production and antioxidant activity of micropropagated *Ceropegia santapaui*. Plant Growth Reg 72:1–15

Chavan, J. J., & Dey, A. (2023). *Zingiber zerumbet* (L.) Roscoe ex Sm.: biotechnological advancements and perspectives. *Applied Microbiology and Biotechnology*, *107*(18), 5613-5625.

Chiou LC, Ling JY, Chang CC (1997) Chinnese herb constituent beta-eudesmol alleviated the electroshock seizures in mice and electrographic seizures in rat hippocampal slices. Neurosci Lett 15:171–174

Chunekar K C., Pandeya G., Bhavaprakash Nighantu. Chaukhamba Sanskrit Santhana, Varanasi, 1979, 45

Chung SY, Jang DS, Han AR, Jang JO, Youngjoo K, Lee HJ, Seo EK (2007) Modulation of P-glycoprotein-mediated resistance by kaemferol derivatives isolated from *Zingiber zerumbet*. Phytother Res 21:565

Dai, D. N., Thang, T. D., Chau, L. T., & Ogunwande, I. A. (2013). Chemical constituents of the root essential oils of *Zingiber* rubens Roxb., and *Zingiber zerumbet* (L.) Smith.

Dambisiya YM, Lee LT (1995) Effects L-NG-nitro arginine methyl ester (L-NAME), L-NG monomethyl arginine (L-NMMA) and L_arginione on the antinociceptive effects of morphine in mice. Exp Clin Pharmacol 17:577–582

Damodaran, N. P., & Dev, S. (1968). Studies in sesquiterpenes—XXXVIII: Structure of humulene epoxide-I and humulene epoxide-II. *Tetrahedron*, *24*(11), 4123-4132.

Das A, Kesari V, Rangan L (2013) Micropropagation and cytogenetic assessment of *Zingiber* species of Northeast India. 3 Biotech 3:471–479

Das Bhowmik, S. S., Basu, A., & Sahoo, L. (2016). Direct shoot organogenesis from rhizomes of medicinal *Zingiber* Alpinia calcarata Rosc. and evaluation of genetic stability by RAPD and ISSR markers. *Journal of crop science and biotechnology*, *19*, 157-165.

DEB, D., Datta, B.K., DEBBARMA, J. and DEB, S., 2016. Ethno-medicinal plants used for herbal medication of jaundice by the indigenous community of Tripura, India. *Biodiversitas Journal of Biological Diversity*, *17*(1).

Dev, S., 1960. Studies in sesquiterpenes – XVI. Zerumbone, a monocyclic sesquiterpene ketone. Tetrahedron 8, 171-180.

Devi, N. B. 2014. *Zingiber*aceae In The Valley Districts of Manipur A Systematic Study.

Devi, N.B., Singh, P.K., Das, A.K., 2014. Ethnomedicinal utilization of *Zingiber*aceae in the valley districts of Manipur. J. Environ. Sci. Toxicol. Food Technol. 8, 21–23

Dewanto, X., Wu, K., Adom, K., Liu, R.H. Thermal processingenhances the nutritional value of tomatoes by increasingtotal antioxidant activity, J. Agric. Food Chem. **2002**, 50, 3010–3014.

Dey A, Nandy S, Nongdam P, Tikendra L, Mukherjee A, Mukherjee S, Pandey DK (2020) Methyl jasmonate and salicylic acid elicit indole alkaloid production and modulate antioxidant defence and biocidal properties in *Rauvolfia serpentina* Benth. ex Kurz. *in vitro* cultures. S Afr J Bot 135:1–7

Dey A, Nongdam P, Nandy S, Mukherjee S, Mukherjee A, Tikendra L, Hazra AK, Pandey DK (2021) Polyamine elicited aristolochic acid production in *in vitro* clonally fidel *Aristolochia indica* L.: an ISSR and RAPD markers and HPTLC based study. S Afr J Bot 140:326–335

Divekar, P., 2023. Botanical pesticides: An eco-friendly approach for Management of Insect Pests. *Acta Scientific Agriculture (ISSN: 2581-365X)*, *7*(2).

Divekar, P.A., Narayana, S., Divekar, B.A., Kumar, R., Gadratagi, B.G., Ray, A., Singh, A.K., Rani, V., Singh, V., Singh, A.K. and Kumar, A., 2022. Plant secondary metabolites as defense tools against herbivores for sustainable crop protection. *International journal of molecular sciences*, *23*(5), p.2690.

Doyle, J.J. and Doyle, J.L., 1987. A rapid DNA isolation procedure for small quantities of fresh leaf tissue. *Phytochemical bulletin.*

Eguchi, A., Kaneko, Y., Murakami, A. and Ohigashi, H., 2007. Zerumbone suppresses phorbol ester-induced expression of multiple scavenger receptor genes in THP-1 human monocytic cells. *Bioscience, biotechnology, and biochemistry*, *71*(4), pp.935- 945.

El Fagie, R.M., Yusoff, N.A., Lim, V., Kamal, N.N.S.N.M. and Samad, N.A., 2021. Anti-cancer and anti-angiogenesis activities of zerumbone isolated from *Zingiber zerumbet*–a systematic review. *Current Research in Nutrition and Food Science Journal*, *9*(2), pp.353-374.

Faridah QZ, Abdelmageed AH, Julia AA, Nor Hafizah R (2011) Efficient *in vitro* regeneration of *Zingiber zerumbet* Smith (a valuable medicinal plant) plantlets from rhizome bud explants. Afr J Biotechnol 10(46):9303–9308

Farnsworth NR, Bunyapraphatsara N (1992) Thai medicinal plants. Prachachou, Bangkok, pp 261–263

Fengnian Y, Okamoto Sh, Harada H, Kazuhisa Y, Norihiko M, Utsumi R (2010) *Zingiber zerumbet* CYP71BA1 catalyzes the conversion of a-humulene to 8-hydroxy-a-humulene in zerumbone biosynthesis. Cell Mol Life Sci 68:1033–1040

Fowsiya, J. and Madhumitha, G., 2020. A review of bioinsecticidal activity and mode of action of plant derived alkaloids. *Research journal of pharmacy and technology*, *13*(2), p.963.

Galvez, C.J., Martin-Cordero, P., Houghton, A.M. Antioxidant activity of methanol extracts obtained from *Plantago* species, J. Agric. Food Chem. 53 (2005) 1927–1933.

George, N.M., Raghav, S.B. and Prasath, D., 2022. Direct *in vitro* regeneration of medicinally important Indian and exotic red-colored ginger (*Zingiber* officinale Rosc.) and genetic fidelity assessment using ISSR and SSR markers. *In vitro Cellular & Developmental Biology-Plant*, *58*(4), pp.551-558.

Ghosh, S., Majumder, P. B., & Mandi, S. S. (2011). Species-specific AFLP markers for identification of *Zingiber* officinale, Z. montanumand *Z. zerumbet* (*Zingiber*aceae). *Genet. Mol. Res*, *10*(1), 218-229.

Girisa, S., Shabnam, B., Monisha, J., Fan, L., Halim, C. E., Arfuso, F., ... & Kunnumakkara, A. B. (2019). Potential of zerumbone as an anti-cancer agent. *Molecules*, *24*(4), 734.

Girisa, S., Shabnam, B., Monisha, J., Fan, L., Halim, C.E., Arfuso, F., Ahn, K.S., Sethi, G. and Kunnumakkara, A.B., 2019. Potential of zerumbone as an anti-cancer agent. *Molecules*, *24*(4), p.734.

Goh S (2019) Improved propagation, maximizing yield and enhancing zerumbone production in *Zingiber zerumbet* (L.) Smith through shading and NPK fertilization. Master's thesis, Universiti Putra Malaysia

Gonzalez-Gonzalez, M., Yerena-Prieto, B.J., Carrera, C., Vázquez-Espinosa, M., González-de-Peredo, A.V., García-Alvarado, M.Á., Palma, M., Rodríguez-Jimenes, G.D.C. and Barbero, G.F., 2023. Optimization of an Ultrasound-Assisted Extraction Method for the Extraction of Gingerols and Shogaols from Ginger (*Zingiber* officinale). *Agronomy*, *13*(7), p.1787.

Gulzar, B., Mujib, A., Malik, M. Q., Mamgain, J., Syeed, R., & Zafar, N. (2020). Plant tissue culture: agriculture and industrial applications. In *Transgenic technology based value addition in plant biotechnology* (pp. 25-49). Academic Press.

Gupta, N., Jain, V., Joseph, M. R., & Devi, S. (2020). A review on micropropagation culture method. *Asian Journal of Pharmaceutical Research and Development*, *8*(1), 86-93.

Hamid D, Ali AM, Rajab NF, Alitheen N, Sirat H, and Bakar AA (2007) Zerumbone causes morphological changes on different types of leukemic cell lines. In: Proceeding of the 24th annual conference of the microscopy society of Thailand, Kasetsart University, Bangkok, Thailand

Han AR, Kim MS, Jeong YH, Lee SK, Seo EK (2005) Cyclooxygenase-2-inhibitory phenylbutanoids from the rhizomes of *Zingiber* cassumunar. Chem Phar Bull 53: 1466–1468

Haque, Md Intesaful, Prashant Kumar Singh, Sandip Ghuge, Anil Kumar, Avinash Chandra Rai, Ajay Kumar, and Arpan Modi. "A general introduction to and background of plant tissue culture: Past, current, and future aspects." In *Advances in Plant Tissue Culture*, pp. 1-30. Academic Press, 2022.

Harada H, Yu F, Okamoto S, Kuzuyama T, Utsumi R, Misawa N (2009) Efficient synthesis of functional isoprenoids from acetoacetate through metabolic pathway-engineered Escherichia coli. Appl Microbiol Biotechnol 81:915–925

Hatano T, Kagawa H, Yasuhara T, Okuda T (1988). Two new flavonoids and other constituents in licorice root: their relative astringency and radical scavenging effects. Chem. Pharm. Bull. 36:2090-2097

Havrilesky LJ, Elbendary A, Hurteau JA, Whittaker RS, Rodriques GC *et al.* (1995) Chemotherapy induced apoptosis in epithelial ovarian cancers. Obst Gynaecol 85:1007–1010

Helen, O.N., Job, A.O. and Oghenebrorhie, O., 2020. Antibiotic and antihelminthic effects of garlic bulbs (Allium sativum) and ginger rhizomes (*Zingiber* officinale) as growth promoters on broiler chickens in the tropics. *Adv. Anim. Vet. Sci*, *8*(10), pp.1019- 1027.

Hoffman AL, Spetner M, Burke M (2002) Redox-regulated mechanism may account for zerumbone's ability to suppress cancer-cell proliferation. Carcinogenesis 23:1961

Hossain ME, Bhattacharjee SC, Islam MDE nayetul. (2005) Chemical investigation on *Zingiber zerumbet*. Frontiers in Natural Product Chemistry (1):185–187

Hsu JY, Yeh CC, Tsay HS (1991) *In vitro* propagation of *Zingiber zerumbet* Smith. J Agric Res China 40(2):171–177

Huang GC, Chien TY, Chen LG, Wang CC. Antitumor effects of zerumbone from *Z. zerumbet* in P-388D1 cells *in vitro* and *in vivo*. Planta Medicine, 2005: 71(3): 219-224

Hunskaar S, Hole K (1987) Preliminary analysis of the antinociceptive activity of Zerumbone. Pain 30:103

Hussain, S., Kapoor, N. and Mahajan, R., 2023. High-frequency Shoot Multiplication and *In vitro* Plantlet Regeneration from Shoot Bud Explants in Curcuma zedoaria Roscoe. *Journal of Herbs, Spices & Medicinal Plants*, *29*(3), pp.262-273.

Ibrahim MY, Abdul AB, Abdel W, Elhassan SI, Alzubairi MN, Syam AS, Elhassan MM (2009) Attenuation of cisplatin induced hepatotoxicity in rats using Zerumbone. Res J Biol Sci 4(7):777–784

Idris ED, Khalid N, Ibrahim H (2007) Production of zerumbone from *in vitro* derived rhizome of *Zingiber zerumbet* for pharmaceutical and cosmeceutical industry. In: 12th biological sciences graduate congress, University of Malaya, 17–19 December 2007

Idris FD, Jali M, Ibrahim H, Khalid N (2009) Establishment of embryogenic cell suspension and field evaluation of regenerants of *Zingiber zerumbet* Smith. Acta Horticulturae 829:p 6

Idris FD, Jalil M, Ibrahim H, Khalid N (2010) Establishment of embryogenic cell suspension and field evaluation of regenerants of *Zingiber zerumbet* Smith. Acta Hortic 829:319–324

Ileke, K.D. and Ogungbite, O.C., 2014. Entomocidal activity of powders and extracts of four medicinal plants against Sitophilus oryzae (L), Oryzaephilus mercator (Faur) and Ryzopertha dominica (Fabr.). *Jordan Journal of Biological Sciences*, *7*(1), pp.57-62.

Islam, J., Zaman, K., Duarah, S., Raju, P.S. and Chattopadhyay, P., 2017. Mosquito repellents: An insight into the chronological perspectives and novel discoveries. *Acta Tropica*, *167*, pp.216-230.

Jang, D. S., Han, A. R., Park, G., Jhon, G. J., & Seo, E. K. (2004). Flavonoids and aromatic compounds from the rhizomes of *Zingiber zerumbet*. *Archives of Pharmacal Research*, *27*, 386-389.

Jang, D.S. and Seo, E.K., 2005. Potentially bioactive two new natural sesquiterpenoids from the rhizomes of *Zingiber zerumbet*. *Archives of Pharmacal Research*, *28*, pp.294-296.

Jantan I, Rafi IAA, Alil J (2005) Platelet activating factor (PAF) receptor binding antagonist activity of Malaysian medicinal plants. Phyto Med 27:799–812

Jose, S., & Thomas, T. D. (2015). High-frequency callus organogenesis, large-scale cultivation and assessment of clonal fidelity of regenerated plants of Curcuma caesia Roxb., an important source of camphor. *Agroforestry Systems*, *89*, 779-788.

Kaçar, Y. A. (2024, April). Somaclonal variation in *in vitro* culture. In *Book of Proceedings* (p. 156).

Kader, G., Nikkon, F., Rashid, M.A. and Yeasmin, T., 2011. Antimicrobial activities of the rhizome extract of *Zingiber zerumbet* Linn. *Asian Pacific journal of tropical biomedicine*, *1*(5), pp.409-412.

Kamaraj, C., Rahuman, A.A., Mahapatra, A., Bagavan, A. and Elango, G., 2010. Insecticidal and larvicidal activities of medicinal plant extracts against mosquitoes. *Parasitology research*, *107*, pp.1337-1349.

Kaur P, Gupta RC, Dey A, Malik T, Pandey DK (2020) Optimization of salicylic acid and chitosan treatment for bitter secoiridoid and xanthone glycosides production in shoot cultures of *Swertia paniculata* using response surface methodology and artificial neural network. BMC Plant Biol 20(1):1–3

Keong YS, Noorjahan BA, Mustafa Sh, Suraini AA, Rahman MA, Abdul MA (2010) Immunomodulatory effects of zerumbone isolated from roots of *Zingiber zerumbet*. Pak J Pharm Sci 23(1):75–82

Keosaeng, K., Songoen, W., Yooboon, T., Bullangpoti, V., & Pluempanupat, W. (2023). Insecticidal activity of isolated gingerols and shogaols from *Zingiber* officinale Roscoe rhizomes against Spodoptera spp.(Lepidoptera: Noctuidae). *Natural Product Research*, *37*(4), 669-674.

Khaskheli, A.J., Ali, M., Baloch, S., Khaskehli, M.I., Rind, M.R. and Zhang, L., 2022. An alternative cost effective method for diminishing contamination severity associated with plant cell and tissue culture. *Global Journal of Research in Science and Technology*, *1*(01), pp.010-021.

Khatun, A., Nasrin, S., & Hossain, M. T. (2003). Large scale multiplication of ginger (*Zingiber* officinale Rosc.) from shoot-tip culture. *J. Biol. Sci*, *3*(1), 59-64.

Kiat TS, Richard P (2006) Screening of selected *Zingiber*aceae extracts for Dengue-2 virus protease inhibitory activities. Sun Acad J 3:1–7

Kimura I (2005) Antiangiogenic activity of b eudesmol *in vitro* and *in vivo*. Eur J Pharmacol 512:105–115

Kinghorn AD, Fransworth NR, Soejarto DD, Cordell GA, Pezzuto JM, Udeani GO, Wani MC, Wall ME, Navarro HA, Kramer RA, Menendez AT, Fairchild CR, Lane KE, Forenza S, Vyas DM, Lams KS, Shu YZ (1997) Novel strategies for the discovery of plant-derived anticancer agents. Pure Appl Chem 71(9):1611–1618

Kirana C, McIntosh GH, Record IR, Jones GP (2003) Antitumour activity of extracts of *Zingiber* aromaticum and its bioactive sesquiterpenoid zerumbone. Nutr Cancer 45:218–225

Kirtikar KR and Basu BD. 1935. *Indian Medicinal Plants.* Vol. III (2nd edn). Basu LM, Allahadad, India. pp.1593-2393.

Kitayama, T. (2011). Attractive reactivity of a natural product, zerumbone. *Bioscience, biotechnology, and biochemistry*, *75*(2), 199-207.

Kitayama, T., Yamamoto, K., Utsumi, R., Takatani, M., Hill, R.K., Kawai, Y., Sawada, S. and Okamoto, T., 2001. Chemistry of zerumbone. 2. Regulation of ring bond cleavage and unique antibacterial activities of zerumbone derivatives. *Bioscience, biotechnology, and biochemistry*, *65*(10), pp.2193-2199.

Koga AY, Beltrame FL, Pereira AV (2016) Several aspects of *Zingiber zerumbet*: a review. Rev Bras Farmacogn 26:385–391

Koshimizu H, Araki T, Takai S, Yokomaku D, Ishikawa Y, Kubota M, Sano S, Hatanaka H, Yamada M (2002) Expression of CD47/integrin-associated protein induces death of cultured cerebral cortical neurons. J Neurochem 82:249–257

Koshimizu K, Ohigashi H, Tokuda H, Kondo A, Yamaguchi K (1988) Screening of edible plants against anti-tumour promoting activity. Cancer Lett 39:24757

Kress, W. J., Prince, L. M., & Williams, K. J. (2002). The phylogeny and a new classification of the gingers (*Zingiber*aceae): evidence from molecular data. *American Journal of Botany*, *89*(10), 1682-1696.

Kress, W. J., Prince, L. M., & Williams, K. J. (2002). The phylogeny and a new classification of the gingers (*Zingiber*aceae): evidence from molecular data. *American Journal of Botany*, *89*(10), 1682-1696.

Kshirsagar P, Umdale S, Chavan J, Gaikwad N (2017) Molecular authentication of medicinal plant, *Swertia chirayita* and its adulterant species. Proc Natl Acad Sci India Sect B Biol Sci 87(1):101–107

Kshirsagar PR, Chavan JJ, Umdale SD, Nimbalkar MS, Dixit GB, Gaikwad NB (2015) Highly efficient *in vitro* regeneration, establishment of callus and cell suspension cultures and RAPD analysis of regenerants of *Swertia lawii* Burkill. Biotech Rep 6:79–84

Kshirsagar PR, Mohite A, Suryawanshi S, Chavan JJ, Gaikwad NB, Bapat VA (2021) Plant regeneration through direct and indirect organogenesis, phyto-molecular profiles, antioxidant properties and swertiamarin production in elicitated cell suspension cultures of *Swertia minor* (Griseb.) Knobl. Plant Cell Tissue Organ Cult 144:383–396

Kumar, N., & Reddy, M. P. (2011). *In vitro* plant propagation: a review. *Journal of forest and environmental science*, *27*(2), 61-72.

Langner E, Greifenberg S, Gruenwald J (1988) Ginger: history and use. Adv Ther 15:25–44

Lim, T. K. (2014). *Zingiber zerumbet.* In *Edible Medicinal and Non Medicinal Plants: Volume 8, Flowers* (pp. 857-876). Dordrecht: Springer Netherlands.

Lowry, O.H., Rosebrough, N.J., Farr, A.L. and Randall, R.J., 1951. Protein measurement with the Folin phenol reagent. *J biol Chem*, *193*(1), pp.265-275.

Madegowda, B.H., Rameshwaran, P., Nagaraju, N.P., Murthy, P.S., 2016. In-vitro mycological activity of essential oil from *Zingiber zerumbet* rhizomes. J. Essent. Oil Res. 28, 81–88.

Madreseh-Ghahfarokhi, S., Pirali, Y., & Dehghani-Samani, A. (2018). The insecticidal and repellent activity of ginger (*Zingiber* officinale) and eucalyptus (Eucalyptus globulus) essential oils against Culex theileri Theobald, 1903 (Diptera: Culicidae). *Annals of parasitology*, *64*(4).

Mansouri, A., Embared, G., Kokkalou, E., Kefalas, P. Phenolic profile and antioxidant activity of the Algerian ripedate palm fruit (*Phoenix dactylifera*), Food Chem. 89 (2005)411–420.

Miranti, M. and Fatiqin, A., 2018, October. Potensi air perasan jahe merah (*Zingiber* officinale Rosc) sebagai Larvasida Aedes aegypti. In *Prosiding Seminar Nasional Sains dan Teknologi Terapan* (Vol. 1).

Miri, S.M., 2020. Micropropagation, callus induction and regeneration of ginger (*Zingiber* officinale Rosc.). *Open agriculture*, *5*(1), pp.75-84.

Mohanty S, Parida R, Kuanar A, Sahoo S, Nayak S (2012) Evaluation of genetic fidelity of *in vitro* propagated shampoo ginger (*Zingiber zerumbet* (L.) Smith) using DNA based markers. J Med Plant Res 6(16):3143–3147

Mohanty S, Parida R, Sahoo S, Nayak S (2014) *In vitro* conservation of nine medicinally and economically important species of *Zingiberaceae* from Eastern India. Proc Natl Acad Sci India Sect B Biol Sci 84:799–803

Murakami A, Hayashi R, Tanaka T, Kwon KH, Ohigashi H, Safitri R (2003) Suppression of dextran sodium sulfateinduced colitis in mice by zerumbone, a subtropical ginger sesquiterpene, and nimesulide: separately and in combination. Biochem Pharmacol 66:1253–1261

Murakami, A., Takahashi, D., Kinoshita, T., Koshimizu, K., Kim, H. W., Yoshihiro, A., ... & Ohigashi, H. (2002). Zerumbone, a Southeast Asian ginger sesquiterpene, markedly suppresses free radical generation, proinflammatory protein production, and cancer cell proliferation accompanied by apoptosis: the α, β-unsaturated carbonyl group is a prerequisite. *Carcinogenesis*, *23*(5), 795-802.

Murakami, A., Takahashi, D., Kinoshita, T., Koshimizu, K., Kim, H.W., Yoshihiro, A., Nakamura, Y., Jiwajinda, S., Terao, J. and Ohigashi, H., 2002. Zerumbone, a Southeast Asian ginger sesquiterpene, markedly suppresses free radical generation, proinflammatory protein production, and cancer cell proliferation accompanied by apoptosis: the α, β-unsaturated carbonyl group is a prerequisite. *Carcinogenesis*, *23*(5), pp.795-802.

Murashige, T. and Skoog, F., 1962. A revised medium for rapid growth and bio assays with tobacco tissue cultures. *Physiologia plantarum*, *15*(3).

Murthy, N. K., Nalini, E., Mageswari, A., Subramanian, P., & Gothandam, K. M. (2022). Chemical Composition and Biological Properties of *Zingiber zerumbet* (L.) Roscoe ex Sm. In *Bioactives and Pharmacology of Medicinal Plants* (pp. 403-416). Apple Academic Press.

Naczk, M., Shahidi, F. Phenolics in cereals, fruits and vegetables:occurrence, extraction and analysis, J. Pharm. Biomed. Anal. 41(2006) 1523–1542

Nakamura Y, Yoshida C, Murakami A, Ohigashi H, Osawa T, Uchida K (2004) Zerumbone, a tropical ginger sesquiterpene, activates phase II drug metabolizing enzymes. FEBS Lett 572(1–3):245–250

Nakamura Y, Yoshida C, Murakami A, Ohigashi H, Osawa T, Uchida K (2004) Zerumbone, a tropical ginger sesquiterpene, activates phase II drug metabolizing enzymes. FEBS Lett 572(1–3):245–250

Nalawade SM, Sagare AP, Lee CY, Kao CL, Tsay HS (2003). Studies on tissue culture of Chinese medicinal plant resources in Taiwan and their sustainable utilization. Bot. Bull. Acad. Sin. 44: 79-98.

Nalawade, S. M., Sagare, A. P., Lee, C. Y., Kao, C. L., & Tsay, H. S. (2003). Studies on tissue culture of Chinese medicinal plant resources in Taiwan and their sustainable utilization. *Bot. Bull. Acad. Sin*, *44*(2), 79-98.

Neeraj M, Chandanamali P, Naoaki F (2009) Hedgehog-Gli signaling pathway inhibitors as anticancer. Agents J Med Chem 52(13):3829–3845

Nigam LC, Levi L (1963a) Zerumbone down-regulates chemokine receptor CXCR4 expression leading to inhibition of CXCL 12-induced I NVASION of breast and pancreatic tumor cells. Can J Chem 41:1726–1730

Nigam, I. C., & Levi, L. (1963). Column and gas chromatographic analysis of oil of wild ginger: identification and estimation of some new constituents. *Canadian journal of Chemistry*, *41*(7), 1726-1730.

Nishino H, Nishino A, Takayasu J, Hasegawa T, Iwashima A, Hirabayashi K, Iwata S, Shibata S (1988) Inhibition of the tumour promoting action of 12-O- tetradecanoylphorbol13-asetate by some oleane-type triterpenoid compounds. Cancer Res 48:5210

Norulaini, N. N., Anuar, O., Omar, A. K. M., AlKarkhi, A. F., Setianto, W. B., Fatehah, M. O., ... & Zaidul, I. S. M. (2009). Optimization of SC–CO2 extraction of zerumbone from *Zingiber zerumbet* (L) Smith. *Food Chemistry*, *114*(2), 702-705.

Norulaini, N. N., Anuar, O., Omar, A. K. M., AlKarkhi, A. F., Setianto, W. B., Fatehah, M. O., ... & Zaidul, I. S. M. (2009). Optimization of SC–CO2 extraction of zerumbone from *Zingiber zerumbet* (L) Smith. *Food Chemistry*, *114*(2), 702-705.

Obara Y (2006) Development of antidementia drugs related to neurotrophic factors. Yakugaku Zasshi 126:747–755

Ohigashi H, Murakami A (2002) Redox-regulated mechanism may account for zerumbone's ability to suppress cancer cell proliferation. Carcinogenesis 23(12):1963

Ormerod MG, Neill CO, Robertson D, Kelland LR, Harrap KR (1996) Cisdiaminedichloroplatinum-induced cell dead through apoptosis in sensitive and resistant human ovarian carcinoma cell lines. Cancer Chemother Pharmacol 37: 463–471

Padalia, R. C., Verma, R. S., Chauhan, A., Singh, V. R., Goswami, P., Singh, S., ... & Darokar, M. P. (2018). *Zingiber zerumbet* (L.) Roscoe ex Sm. from northern India: Potential source of zerumbone rich essential oil for antiproliferative and antibacterial applications. *Industrial Crops and Products*, *112*, 749-754.

Padalia, R.C., Verma, R.S., Chauhan, A. and Chanotiya, C.S., 2013. Changes in aroma profiles of 11 Indian Ocimum taxa during plant ontogeny. *Acta Physiologiae Plantarum*, *35*, pp.2567-2587.

Pant, B. (2014). Application of plant cell and tissue culture for the production of phytochemicals in medicinal plants. In *Infectious Diseases and Nanomedicine II: First International Conference (ICIDN–2012), Dec. 15-18, 2012, Kathmandu, Nepal* (pp. 25-39). Springer India.

Paramita, A., Wibowo, I., & Insanu, M. (2021). A study of genus *Zingiber*: The role of condiments in science. *Current Research on Biosciences and Biotechnology*, *3*(1), 186-195.

Pawar, N. V., Pai, S. R., Nimbalkar, M. S., & Dixit, G. B. (2015). RP-HPLC analysis of phenolic antioxidant compound 6-gingerol from *in vitro* cultures of *Zingiber* officinale Roscoe. *Plant Science Today*, *2*(1), 24-28.

Peredo, E.L., Revilla, M.Á. and Arroyo-García, R., 2006. Assessment of genetic and epigenetic variation in hop plants regenerated from sequential subcultures of organogenic calli. *Journal of Plant Physiology*, *163*(10), pp.1071-1079.

Peri LM (1980) Medicinal plants of East and South East Asia. Attributed properties and uses. MIT press, Cambridge

Permadi, N., Nurzaman, M., Alhasnawi, A.N., Doni, F. and Julaeha, E., 2023. Managing lethal browning and microbial contamination in Musa spp. tissue culture: Synthesis and perspectives. *Horticulturae*, *9*(4), p.453.

Perrin, A., Schaffner, F., Christe, P. and Glaizot, O., 2023. Relative effects of urbanisation, deforestation, and agricultural development on mosquito communities. *Landscape Ecology*, *38*(6), pp.1527-1536.

Poonsapaya P, Kraisintu K (1993). Micropropagation of *Zingiber* cassumanar. Acta Hortic., 344: 557-564.

Prajapati, N. D., Purohit, S. S., Sharma, A. K., & Kumar, T. (2003). Medicinal plants. *Agrobios published company, 3rd edition, India, 353*.

Prakash, R. O., Rabinarayan, A., & Kumar, M. S. (2011). *Zingiber zerumbet* (L.) Sm., a reservoir plant for therapeutic uses: A review. *International Journal of Research in Ayurveda and Pharmacy*, *2*, 1-22.

Preshahdin, N.A., Jani, N.A. and Iberahim, R., 2023. Phytochemicals and antibacterial activity of *Zingiber zerumbet* growing in Negeri Sembilan, Malaysia. *Journal of Science and Mathematics Letters*, *11*(1), pp.20-29.

Prieto, P., Pineda, M., Aguilar, M. Spectrophotometric quantitationof antioxidant capacity through the formation of a phospho-molybdenum complex: specific application to the determinationof vitamin E, Anal. Biochem. 269 (1999) 337–341.

Rahman, H. S., Rasedee, A., Chartrand, M. S., Othman, H. H., Yeap, S. K., & Namvar, F. (2014). Zerumbone induces G2/M cell cycle arrest and apoptosis via mitochondrial pathway in Jurkat cell line. *Natural Product Communications*, *9*(9), 1934578X1400900904.

Rakkimuthu, R., Jacob, J., & Aravinthan, K. M. (2011). *In vitro* micropropagation of Alpinia zerumbet Variegate, an important medicinal plant, through rhizome bud explants. *Res Biotechnol*, *2*(1), 7-10.

Ramaswami, S.K., Bhattacharyya, S.C., 1962. Terpenoids – XXXI. Isolation of humulene monoxide and humulene dioxide. Tetrahedron 18, 575-579.

Ramzan, M. and Zeshan, B., 2023. Assessment of the phytochemical analysis and antimicrobial potentials of *Zingiber zerumbet*. *Molecules*, *28*(1), p.409.

Rana, V.S., Ahluwalia, V., Shakil, N.A. and Prasad, L., 2017. Essential oil composition, antifungal, and seedling growth inhibitory effects of zerumbone from *Zingiber zerumbet* Smith. *Journal of essential oil research*, *29*(4), pp.320-329.

Ranemma, M., Reddy, S.K. 2017. Phytochemical Investigation Study of *Curcuma caesia* Roxb Different Geographical Regions (Delhi and Orissa) of India. *IOSR Journal of Biotechnology and Biochemistry* 3(1): 23-26

Ranemma, M., Reddy, S.K. 2017. Genetic Diversity and Similarity Studies in Different Accessions of *Curcuma caesia* Roxb. by RAPD Analysis. *Trends in Biosciences*, 10(27): 5684-5689.

Rao, K.S., Haran, R.H. and Rajpoot, V.S., 2022. Value addition: A novel strategy for quality enhancement of medicinal and aromatic plants. *Journal of Applied Research on Medicinal and Aromatic Plants*, *31*, p.100415.

Rasmos S, Alia M, Bravo L, Goya L (2005) Comparative effects of food derived polyphenols on the viability and apoptosis of a human hepatoma cell line (HepG2). J Agric Food Chem 53:1271–1280

Rawat A, Kholiya S, Chauhan A, Venkatesha KT, Kumar D, Upadhyay RK, Padalia RC (2024) Chemical variability on *Zingiber zerumbet* (L.) Roscoe ex Sm. essential oil with respect to different comminution methods. Biochem Syst Ecol 106:104574

Rawat, A., Kholiya, S., Chauhan, A., Srivastava, D., Pal, A., Verma, R.S., Chanotiya, C.S. and Padalia, R.C., 2024. Effect of post-harvest drying period on the chemical composition of *Zingiber zerumbet* Sm. Rhizomes essential oil and its biological activities. *Physiology and Molecular Biology of Plants*, pp.1-11.

Reddy, K.S., Rao, K.N.V., Saikrishna, J., Mahendra, K. and Mani, P., 2024. A review on the medicinal plant *Zingiber zerumbet* phytochemical composition, traditional uses, and potential health benefits.

Roosterman D, Goerge T, Schneider SW, Bunnett NW, Steinhoff M (2006) Neuronal control of skin function: the skin as a neuroimmunoendocrine organ. Physiol Rev 86:1309–1379

Rosentrater, K.A., 2022. Insects in grains: identification, damage, and detection. In *Storage of cereal grains and their products* (pp. 607-646). Woodhead Publishing.

Rout, K. K., Mishra, S. K., & Sherma, J. (2009). Development and validation of an HPTLC method for analysis of zerumbone, the anticancer marker from *Zingiber zerumbet*. *Acta Chromatographica*, *21*(3), 443-452.

Sahu, A. K., Panda, C., & Nayak, B. S. (2018). Determination of phytochemical and anthelmintic activity of rhizome of *Zingiber zerumbet*. *J Pharm Adv Res*, *1*, 399-402.

Sarker, S.S., Ahmed, K.M., Tanny, T., Nasrin, S., Rahman, A.M., Das, K.C. and Alam, I., 2023. Molecular identification and high fidelity micropropagation of shell ginger (Alpinia zerumbet). *All Life*, *16*(1), p.2169960.

Sathishkumar, P., Hemalatha, S., Arulkumar, M., Ravikumar, R., Yusoff, A. R. M., Hadibarata, T., & Palvannan, T. (2015). Curcuminoid Extraction from Turmeric (C urcuma Longa L.): Efficacy of Bromine-Modified Curcuminoids Against Food Spoilage Flora. *Journal of Food Biochemistry*, *39*(3), 325-333.

Sharifah Sakinah, S. A., Tri Handayani, S., & Azimahtol Hawariah, L. P. (2007). Zerumbone induced apoptosis in liver cancer cells via modulation of Bax/Bcl-2 ratio. *Cancer cell international*, *7*, 1-11.

Sharifah Sakinah, S. A., Tri Handayani, S., & Azimahtol Hawariah, L. P. (2007). Zerumbone induced apoptosis in liver cancer cells via modulation of Bax/Bcl-2 ratio. *Cancer cell international*, *7*, 1-11.

Sharifi-Rad, M., Varoni, E. M., Salehi, B., Sharifi-Rad, J., Matthews, K. R., Ayatollahi, S. A., ... & Rigano, D. (2017). Plants of the genus *Zingiber* as source of antimicrobial agents: from tradition to pharmacy.

Sharim, M. and Shamsiah, A., 2021. Detection of changes in growth, yield and genetic variation using RAPD markers among M1V2 and M1V3 generations of irradiated ginger (*Zingiber* officinale Roscoe). *Food Research*, *5*(4), pp.74-82.

Sharma, T. R., & Singh, B. M. (1995). *In vitro* microrhizome production in *Zingiber* officinale Rosc. *Plant cell reports*, *15*(3), 274-277.

Shcherbakova, L.A., 2019. Fungicide resistance of plant pathogenic fungi and their chemosensitization as a tool to increase anti-disease effects of triazoles and strobilurines. *Sel'skokhozyaistvennaya Biol*, *54*, pp.875-891.

Shinija K, Preethi TP, Rakhi KP, Sabu M, Madhusoodanan PV, Benjamin S (2009) Micropropagation and chemical profiling of *Zingiber zerumbet*. J Trop Med Plant 10(1):55–59

Shofiyani, A., Suwarto, Suprayogi and Yuniaty, A., 2023. Growth characteristics and production of bioactive compounds in aromatic ginger (Kaempferia galanga) callus under photoperiod and auxin treatments.

Shukla, R., Singh, P., Prakash, B., Kumar, A., Mishra, P.K. and Dubey, N.K., 2011. Efficacy of essential oils of Lippia alba (Mill.) NE Brown and Callistemon lanceolatus (Sm.) Sweet and their major constituents on mortality, oviposition and feeding behaviour of pulse beetle, Callosobruchus chinensis L. *Journal of the Science of Food and Agriculture*, *91*(12), pp.2277-2283.

Sidahmed, H. M. A., Hashim, N. M., Abdulla, M. A., Ali, H. M., Mohan, S., Abdelwahab, S. I., ... & Vadivelu, J. (2015). Antisecretory, gastroprotective, antioxidant and anti-Helicobcter pylori activity of zerumbone from *Zingiber zerumbet* (L.) Smith. *PloS one*, *10*(3), e0121060.

Sidahmed, H.M.A., Hashim, N.M., Abdulla, M.A., Ali, H.M., Mohan, S., Abdelwahab, S.I., Taha, M.M.E., Fai, L.M. and Vadivelu, J., 2015. Antisecretory, gastroprotective, antioxidant and anti-*Helicobacter pylori* activity of zerumbone from *Zingiber zerumbet* (L.) Smith. *PloS one*, *10*(3), p.e0121060.

Singh CB, Nongalleima K, Brojendrosingh S, Ningombam S, Lokendrajit N, Singh LW (2012) Biological and chemical properties of *Zingiber zerumbet* Smith: a review. Phytochem Rev 11:113–125

Singh, N., Choudhury, D. R., Singh, A. K., Kumar, S., Srinivasan, K., Tyagi, R. K., ... & Singh, R. (2013). Comparison of SSR and SNP markers in estimation of genetic diversity and population structure of Indian rice varieties. *PloS one*, *8*(12), e84136.

Singh, Y. P., Girisa, S., Banik, K., Ghosh, S., Swathi, P., Deka, M., ... & Kunnumakkara, A. B. (2019). Potential application of zerumbone in the prevention and therapy of chronic human diseases. *Journal of Functional Foods*, *53*, 248-258.

Singh, Y.P., Girisa, S., Banik, K., Ghosh, S., Swathi, P., Deka, M., Padmavathi, G., Kotoky, J., Sethi, G., Fan, L. and Mao, X., 2019. Potential application of zerumbone in the prevention and therapy of chronic human diseases. *Journal of Functional Foods*, *53*, pp.248-258.

Siregar, R.S., Bangun, I.H., Saleh, A., Silalahi, M., Apriyanti, I., Kamaludin, M. and Abogazia, A.H., 2024. Exploring Ginger as Botanical Pesticides for Sustainable Maize Protection, Economic Growth, and Landscape Planning Strategies for Maize in North Sumatra, Indonesia. *ARPHA Preprints*, *5*, p.e122499.

Sirirugsa, P. (1999). Thai *Zingiber*aceae: species diversity and their uses. *Pure Appl Chem*, *70*(11), 1-8.

Sirirugsa, P. (1999). Thai *Zingiber*aceae: species diversity and their uses. *Pure Appl Chem*, *70*(11), 1-8.

Somchit MN, Shukriyah MH (2005) Anti-inflammatory property of ethanol and water extracts of *Z. zerumbet*. Indian Pharmacol 35:181–182

Somchit, M. N., & Shukriyah, M. N. (2003). Anti inflammatory property of ethanol and water extracts of *Zingiber zerumbet*. *Indian Journal of Pharmacology*, *35*(3), 181- 182.

Soroush, A., Pourhossein, S., Hosseingholizadeh, D., Hjazi, A., Shahhosseini, R., Kavoosi, H., Kermanshahi, N., Behnamrad, P., Ghavamikia, N., Dadashpour, M. and Karkon Shayan, S., 2024. Anti-cancer potential of zerumbone in cancer and glioma: current trends and future perspectives. *Medical Oncology*, *41*(5), p.125.

Soumya, T., Jayasree, P. R., & Manish Kumar, P. R. (2023). *Zingiber*aceae Plants: A Cornucopia of Promising Chemotherapeuticals for Cancer Cure. *Bioprospecting of Tropical Medicinal Plants*, 427-462.

Stanly C, Bhatt A, Ali HMD (2011) Evaluation of free radical scavenging activity and total phenolic content in the petiole-derived callus cultures of *Zingiber zerumbet* Smith. J Med Plant Res 5(11):2210–2217

Stanly C, Keng CL (2007) Micropropagation of *Curcuma zedoaria* Rosc. and *Zingiber zerumbet* Smith. Biotechnol 6(4):555–560

Stanly, C., & Keng, C. L. (2007). Micropropagation of Curcuma zedoaria roscoe and *Zingiber zerumbet* smith. *Biotechnology*, *6*(4), 555-560.

Sulaiman MR, Perimal EK, Zakaria ZA, Mokhtar F, Lajis NH, Israf DA (2009) Preliminary analysis of the antinociceptive activity of zerumbone. Fitoterpia 80:230–232

Sun, B., Richardo-Da-Silvia, J.M., Spranger, I. Critical factors ofvanillin assay for catechins and proanthocyanidins, J. Agric. FoodChem. **1998**, 46, 4267–4274.

Supinya T, Sanan S (2007) Antiallergic activity of some selected plants in the *Zingiber*aceae family. J Ethnopharmacol 109:535–538

Suthisut, D., Fields, P. G., & Chandrapatya, A. (2011). Contact toxicity, feeding reduction, and repellency of essential oils from three plants from the ginger family

(*Zingiber*aceae) and their major components against Sitophilus zeamais and Tribolium castaneum. *Journal of economic entomology*, *104*(4), 1445-1454.

Swapana, N., Lokendrajit, N., Warjeet, S., Laitonjam, C., Singh, B. Antioxidant activities of the rhizomes of different *Zingiber*aceae plants of north-east India, Asian J. Biol. Life Sci. 2 (2013) 19–22.

Szabolcs A, Tiszlavicz L, Kaszaki J, Posa A, Berko A, Varga IS, Boros I, Szuts V, Lonovics J (2007) Zerumbone exerts a beneficial effect on inflammatory parameters of cholecystokinin octapeptide-induced experimental pancreatitis but fails to improve histology. Pancrease 35(30):249–255

Taha MME, Abdula BA, Abdullah R, Ibrahimc TAT, Abdelwahaba SI, Mohana S (2010) Potential chemoprevention of diethylnitrosamine-initiated and 2-acetylaminofluorene-promoted hepatocarcinogenesis by zerumbone from the rhizomes of the subtropical ginger (*Zingiber zerumbet*). Chem Biol Interact 186(3):295–305

Taha, M. M. E., Abdul, A. B., Abdullah, R., Ibrahim, T. A. T., Abdelwahab, S. I., & Mohan, S. (2010). Potential chemoprevention of diethylnitrosamine-initiated and 2-acetylaminofluorene-promoted hepatocarcinogenesis by zerumbone from the rhizomes of the subtropical ginger (*Zingiber zerumbet*). *Chemico-Biological Interactions*, *186*(3), 295-305.

Takada Y, Murakami A, Agarwal BB (2005) Zerumbone abolishes NF-kappa B and I Kappa Balpha kinase activation leading to suppression of anti-apoptotic and metastatic gene expression, upregulation of apoptosis and down regulation of invasion. Oncogene 17:122–130

Talla, S.K., Bagari, P., Manga, S., Aileni, M. and Mamidala, P., 2022. Comparative study of micropropagated plants of Grand Naine banana during *in vitro* regeneration and *ex vitro* acclimatization. *Biocatalysis and Agricultural Biotechnology*, *42*, p.102325.

Talla, S.K., Madam, E., Manga, S., Aileni, M. and Mamidala, P., 2019. Efficient TDZ- induced regeneration from capitulum explants of *Gerbera jamesonii* Bolus ex Hooker F.-an ornamental plant with high aesthetic value. *Plant Biosystems-An International Journal Dealing with all Aspects of Plant Biology*, *153*(5), pp.679-685.

Tan, E.S., Aminah, A., Khalid, H.M., Maskat, M.Y., Ghani, M.A. Antioxidant properties of three banana cultivars (*Musa acuminata*'*Berangan*', '*Mas*' and '*Raja*') extracts, Sains Malays. 41, 2012. 319–324.

Tanaka T, Shimizu M, Kohno H, Yoshitani S, Hideki M (2001) Chemopreventive of azoxymethane-induced rat abberant crypt foci by dietary zerubone isolated from *Zingiber zerumbet*. Life Sci 69:1935–1945

Tandon B, Anand U, Alex BK, Kaur P, Nandy S, Shekhawat MS, Sanyal R, Pandey DK, Koshy EP, Dey A 2021. Statistical optimization of *in vitro* callus induction of wild and cultivated varieties of *Mucuna pruriens* L.(DC.) using response surface methodology and assessment of L-Dopa biosynthesis. Ind Crops Prod 169:113626

Tandon, V., Yadav, A. K., Roy, B., Das, B. 2011. Phytochemicals as cure of worm infections in traditional medicine systems. *Emerging trends in zoology*, *16*, 351-378.

Thavara, U., Tawatsin, A., Bhakdeenuan, P., Wongsinkongman, P., Boonruad, T., Bansiddhi, J., Chavalittumrong, P., Komalamisra, N., Siriyasatien, P. and Mulla, M.S., 2007. Repellent activity of essential oils against cockroaches (Dictyoptera: Blattidae, Blattellidae, and Blaberidae) in Thailand. *Southeast Asian J Trop Med Public Health*, *38*(4), pp.663-673.

Tikendra, L., Potshangbam, A.M., Dey, A., Devi, T.R., Sahoo, M.R., Nongdam, P. 2021. RAPD, ISSR, and SCoT markers based genetic stability assessment of micropropagated *Dendrobium fimbriatum* Lindl. var. *oculatum* Hk. f.-an important endangered orchid. Physiol Mol Biol Plants 27:341–357

Tushar, S.B., Sarma, G.C., Rangan, L., 2010. Ethnomedical uses of *Zingiberaceous* plants of Northeast India. J. Ethnopharmacol. 132, 286-296

Uma, E., Muthukumar, T. 2014. Comparative root morphological anatomy of *Zingiberaceae*. *Systematics and Biodiversity*, *12*(2), 195-209.

Venkateshgoud, V., Reddy, S.K. 2024. Genetic analysis of dragon fruit *Selenicereus species*. *World Journal of Pharmaceutical Research.* 13 (7): 614-622

Voravuthikunchai, S.P., Limsuwan, S., Supapol, O. and Subhadhirasakul, S., 2006. Antibacterial activity of extracts from family *Zingiberaceae* against foodborne pathogens. *Journal of food safety*, *26*(4), pp.325-334.

Xian, M., Ito, K., Nakazato, T. 2007. Zerumbone, a bioactive sesquiterpene, induces G2 /M cell cycle arrest and apoptosis in leukemia cells via a Fas- and mitochondria mediated pathway. Cancer Sci 98:118–126

Yob, N.J., Jofrry, S.M., Affandi, M., The, L., Salleh, M., and Zakaria, Z. 2011. *Z. zerumbet* (L.) Smith: a review of its ethnomedicinal, chemical, and pharmacological uses. Evid. Based Complement. Alternat. Med., 2011: 543216

Yu, F., Okamto, S., Nakasone, K., Adachi, K., Matsuda, S., Harada, H., ... & Utsumi, R. 2008. Molecular cloning and functional characterization of α-humulene synthase, a possible key enzyme of zerumbone biosynthesis in shampoo ginger (*Zingiber zerumbet* Smith). *Planta*, *227*, 1291-1299.

Zaka, S.M., Iqbal, N., Saeed, Q., Akrem, A., Batool, M., Khan, A.A., Anwar, A., Bibi, M., Azeem, S., Bibi, R. and Khan, K.A., 2019. Toxic effects of some insecticides, herbicides, and plant essential oils against Tribolium confusum Jacquelin du val (Insecta: Coleoptera: Tenebrionidae). *Saudi journal of biological sciences*, *26*(7), pp.1767-1771.

Zakaria, Z., Mohamad, A.A.S., Chear, C,T., Wong, Y.Y., Israf, D.A., Sulaiman, M.R. 2010. Anti-inflammatory and antinociceptive activities of *Zingiber zerumbet* methanol extract in experimental model systems. Med Princ Pract 19:287–294

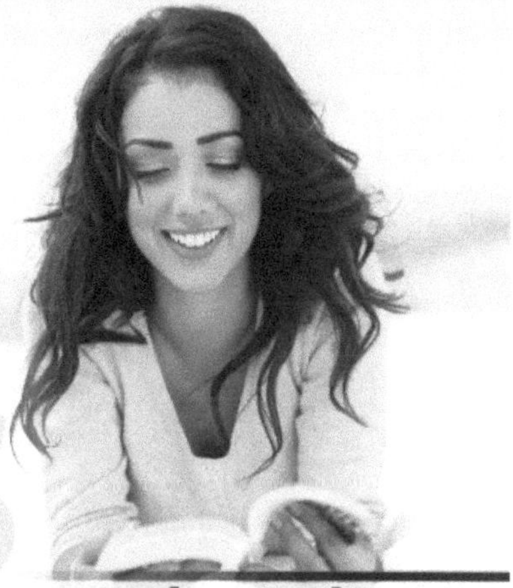

Druck:
CPI Druckdienstleistungen GmbH
im Auftrag der
Kolibri 360 GmbH
Ferdinand-Jühlke-Str. 7
99095 Erfurt

FSC
www.fsc.org
MIX
Papier | Fördert gute Waldnutzung
FSC® C083411

Kolibri 360 GmbH
Ferdinand-Jühlke-Straße 7
99095 Erfurt, Deutschland
produktsicherheit@kolibri360.de